Praise for *A Happy, Healthy Mom*

"So many mothers carry a quiet, persistent sense of not being enough. *A Happy, Healthy Mom* is a deeply needed offering—a reminder that true caregiving must include ourselves. With wisdom and practical guidance, this book shows how stress, depletion, and isolation take root—and how, with care, we can restore balance. An empowering and reassuring guide, it supports mothers in reconnecting with their innate resilience, vitality, and capacity for joy."

—Tara Brach, PhD, author of *Radical Acceptance* and *Radical Compassion*

"This book offers thoughtful, compassionate support for mothers navigating the very real demands of raising children while also trying to care for themselves. With warmth and practicality, it reminds us that tending to a parent's well-being is not a luxury; it's foundational to the health of the whole family. A reassuring and encouraging resource for any mom who has ever felt overwhelmed or depleted."

—Tina Payne Bryson, PhD, *New York Times* bestselling coauthor of *The Whole-Brain Child*

"*A Happy, Healthy Mom* is a compassionate and much-needed guide for the realities of modern motherhood. Grounded in science and real-life experience, it helps mothers restore their energy, health, and emotional balance without judgment or self-blame. Rather than asking moms to do more, this book offers practical, realistic ways to feel supported and well—so they can truly thrive, not just get through the day."

—Kristin Neff, PhD, author of *Self-Compassion* and *Fierce Self-Compassion*

"This indispensable book is both a rallying call for nurturing motherhood, the most essential function in human life, and also a thoughtful primer for moms and those who support them. Wise, practical, and in places uproariously witty, *A Happy, Healthy Mom* is a gift to the generations, present and future."

—Gabor Maté, MD, *New York Times* bestselling author of *The Myth of Normal*

"For mothers who feel as though they are swimming upstream, this book offers both recognition and relief. The authors illuminate Depleted Mother Syndrome with clarity, compassion, and deep practical wisdom, and offer a treasure trove of strategies for addressing stress at the personal, physical, and relational levels. Written in a voice that is warm, wise, and deeply reassuring, this is a book readers will return to again and again. I highly recommend it for mothers—and for women in any caregiving role."

—Diana Divecha, PhD, assistant clinical professor at Yale Child Study Center

"As a mother and clinical psychologist, I believe one of the most important questions we can ask is: How do we help mothers use their precious energy in ways that sustain both their well-being and their families? *A Happy, Healthy Mom* answers that question with wisdom, compassion, and a deeply holistic, science-informed view of motherhood. It is a powerful reminder that caring for mothers is the wisest use of our energy. Healthy moms change the world."

—Diana Hill, PhD, author of *Wise Effort: How to Focus Your Genius Energy on What Matters Most*

"*A Happy, Healthy Mom* is a thoughtful, compassionate, and unusually comprehensive guide to the long stretch of motherhood that begins after the early postpartum spotlight fades. Without sentimentality or simplistic advice, Rick Hanson, Jan Hanson, and Ricki Pollycove take seriously the ways chronic stress, physical depletion, and relational strain can shape a mother's life—and they offer grounded, practical help for easing that burden. There is a humane quality to this deeply useful book that will help mothers feel both understood and better equipped for the years of raising young children. Strongly recommended."

—Steven C. Hayes, PhD, foundation professor emeritus of psychology at the University of Nevada, Reno; originator of Acceptance and Commitment Therapy (ACT); and author of *A Liberated Mind*

A Happy, Healthy MOM

Also by Rick Hanson, PhD, Jan Hanson, LAc, and Ricki Pollycove, MD

Mother Nurture

Also by Rick Hanson, PhD

Buddha's Brain

Just One Thing

Hardwiring Happiness

Resilient

Neurodharma

Making Great Relationships

Also by Ricki Pollycove, MD

The Pocket Guide to Bioidentical Hormones

A Happy, Healthy MOM

Your Guide to Less Stress, Better Teamwork, and More Joy on the Journey

RICK HANSON, PHD, JAN HANSON, LAC,

AND RICKI POLLYCOVE, MD, with RENEE BRNA

BENBELLA

BenBella Books, Inc.
Dallas, TX

This book is for informational purposes only. It is not intended to serve as a substitute for professional medical advice. The author and publisher specifically disclaim any and all liability arising directly or indirectly from the use of any information contained in this book. A healthcare professional should be consulted regarding your specific medical situation. Any product mentioned in this book does not imply endorsement of that product by the author or publisher.

BENBELLA

BenBella Books, Inc.
8080 N. Central Expressway
Suite 1700
Dallas, TX 75206
benbellabooks.com
Send feedback to feedback@benbellabooks.com

Printed in the United States of America
10 9 8 7 6 5 4 3 2 1

Library of Congress Control Number: 2026011125
ISBN 9781637749333 (trade paperback)
ISBN 9781637749340 (electronic)

Copyediting by Karen Wise
Proofreading by Marissa Wold Uhrina and Sarah Vostok
Indexing by WordCo. Indexing Services
Text design and composition by PerfecType, Nashville, TN
Cover design by Stephanie Veillon
Cover image by Stephanie Veillon and © Adobe Stock / artbesouro and lyudinka
Printed by Lake Book Manufacturing

To our parents—
Helen and William Hanson
Dorothy and Ray Emge
Rosalyn and Myron Pollycove
Susan and Craig Brna

And to our children—Laurel, Forrest, Leah, Evelyn, and Max

CONTENTS

INTRODUCTION

by Jan Hanson, LAC

Motherhood is a very personal, very individual experience, yet you may have had people who don't know you at all tell you how to do some part of it, from strangers on the street to professionals in print—like us. So I felt you ought to know where we're coming from, and why we wrote this book.

Being a mother has been the most wonderful, extraordinary experience of my life, and I wouldn't trade it for anything! But by the time our son was three and his baby sister was a few months old, I had been working hard and living with stress for so long, with so little replenishment coming back in, that it all caught up with me. I kept going every day, but I had become very drained, both physically and emotionally.

I saw variations on the same theme with my friends who were mothers. Some, like me, had hit bottom. Others felt their health and well-being were worsening, though reserves remained inside. Many were still sailing along, yet they were definitely frazzled and tired.

But every mom I knew was surprised by the impact of becoming a parent, and wished she knew more about coping with it. Many of us felt let down by our partners, who weren't helping enough at home or couldn't seem to understand what we were going through. And a number of women, including myself, had developed nagging problems that began soon after we had children—such as intensified hormonal ups and downs, depressed mood, or disturbances in the digestive tract—and these seemed impossible to get rid of while we were so busy and stressed. We told each other this was not how motherhood was supposed to be, but we didn't know what to do about it.

Neither, it seemed, did anyone else. During our pregnancies and for a few months postpartum, we received excellent care, but by our babies' first birthdays, we had dropped off the radar of the medical system.

It's as if raising a family has no lasting effects on a woman's health and well-being. Of course, this is not the real truth.

Over time, Rick and I began to realize that every mother needs to lower her stresses and replenish her body—and many would also like to have a strong relationship with a partner—or else she is likely to become physically depleted, which was exactly what had happened to me.

In retrospect, it seemed obvious: Moms give so much nurturance to others that they need to receive it as well. In order to find out what mothers needed, Rick and I studied the research on mothers, talked with leading clinicians, asked moms what had worked for them, drew on our professional experience, and tried different things with me. We applied what we learned to the women in our practices and saw how they benefited.

Along the way, we looked for a book that could guide us, but there wasn't much available past the first year postpartum—and the deepest lows of depletion seem to hit most mothers two or more years after their baby was born. So we resolved to create a book ourselves. Rick has written most of it, and we've also had the good fortune to work with Dr. Ricki Pollycove, an expert on women's health—and mother herself—whose sound medical judgment and warmhearted understanding of moms and their families are woven throughout these pages.

More than anything, we wrote the book Ricki and I wished we'd had when we became mothers! Our focus is on those years when children are especially young, before starting first grade, because that's usually when the demands on a mother are the greatest. Since there already are many excellent books on the first few postpartum months, we emphasize the many months and years that stretch ahead after that. We address your mind, body, and relationships because each of these aspects of your life is affected by motherhood. We offer a spectrum of methods to improve your health and well-being, from mild to intensive, and conventional to alternative, since individual mothers need and want different things.

Chapter 1 gives an overview of how bearing and rearing children wear on women, and it tells how three mothers successfully used the basic "happy, healthy mom" prescription: *Lower the demands on you, increase your resources, and build up your resilience.* Chapters 2 and 3 present ways to cope with stress and manage the thornier emotions that often intensify with parenthood, including sadness, anxiety, shame, and anger. Chapters 4 and 5 explain how to keep your body well in the first place, and what to do if it's getting depleted. Chapters 6, 7, and 8 focus on building teamwork and intimacy with a partner. Chapter 9 covers the practical issue that's a big stressor for many women today: how to juggle motherhood and work. Several appendixes address topics such as how to get the most out of working with your health care providers. And if you are interested in the scientific studies we've relied on, the reference notes are posted on our website, www.ahappyhealthymom.com, where you will find additional information about nurturing yourself and your family. In general, feel free to jump ahead to topics that are pressing and come back later to earlier sections of the book.

Throughout, you'll find many suggestions for improving your health and well-being. Some are specific to mothers, while others are general methods that we've adapted to women raising children. We don't expect you to try them all, just the ones that suit you—and feel free to adapt those to your own situation. Please know that our general statements will not apply to everyone, and that this book is no substitute for professional care. If you have an acute condition of any kind, we urge you to consult immediately with a licensed professional.

Before we dive in, I'd like to create a context, since motherhood can be an emotionally charged, even controversial subject these days:

- Nurturing a mom doesn't mean doing less for her kids. When mothers improve their health and well-being, they are more able to be highly loving and skillful parents. We've tried to answer the question that gripped us soon after our first child was born: How can a mother get what *she* needs to keep giving her children what *they* need, year after year after year?
- Mother nurture is not just an issue for biological parents. Women who adopt children are as affected by overwork, stress, and poor replenishment as any other mother.
- Healthy and happy families take many forms, and we sure don't think that there's only one right way to do it. This said, an important potential source of support for a mother is teamwork and intimacy with a co-parent, whether that's the biological father of her children or someone else. If you're not currently involved with a co-parent, you'll still find ideas and tools in chapters 6, 7, and 8 that will be useful in other kinds of relationships. Some mothers are raising their children with another woman, but for simplicity—and with an apology—we'll generally use the masculine pronoun to refer to a mother's partner. We also use the terms *marriage* and *partnership*, as well as *husband*, *spouse*, and *partner*, interchangeably.
- Many of the factors that wear on mothers originate in America's culture, legal and health care systems, and economy, as

well as in our long history of sexism and racism. Changes in these would benefit mothers greatly (please see the afterword), but that's a larger subject than our focus in this book.

- Research on how motherhood affects a woman's long-term health and well-being has been sadly limited. Still, we've done a deep dive into the available research. To keep things readable, we've chosen to use Reference Notes linked to specific words or phrases, and these are posted at the book's website: www.ahappyhealthymom.com, where you will find many additional free guides, meditations, and other resources.
- There are large individual differences among mothers, fathers, children, and families. So when we talk about "mothers" or "fathers," we mean the midrange of a group seen with less than perfect clarity. This is not academic hairsplitting, but concern for the unique truth of each particular person.
- We are middle-aged, middle-class, and white—and many mothers are not. Most of the mothers we know come from backgrounds that are similar to ours, and our suggestions will not apply to everyone. We hope that others will be able to build on our beginning to help *all* of the women who are bearing and rearing our precious children.

So much of what we have learned has come from other mothers and fathers. Parents are all in this together. Our warmest hope is that you can create a wonderful home for yourself and your family. We wish you the best!

PART ONE

Understanding the Challenges of Motherhood

CHAPTER ONE

Refilling Your Cupboard

A baby is an inestimable blessing and bother.

Mark Twain

Nothing changes your life like a child, and there's really no way to prepare for it. Suddenly you're working all the time, hitting the red line on stress, and you look around and wonder, *Where's the support?* In our practices, we see mothers every day who feel frayed around the edges, let down by their partners, and worn out—or worse. Some have developed serious physical or marital problems since becoming a mom. Many women feel that it's their fault or that they must be the only one who can't handle the strain. They figure that feeling overwhelmed just comes with the territory.

Well, we're here to tell you that you're not to blame and you're not alone. What's more, there are plenty of practical things you can do that will help you feel better and bring more teamwork and closeness into your relationship with your partner.

In this chapter, you'll read about three women who came to us for treatment and exactly what they did to improve their health and well-being. Just as we hope to do for you over the course of this book, we helped each one of these mothers to:

- Lower the demands on her.
- Increase her resources.
- Build up her resilience.

That's what it takes to be a happy, healthy mom.

And you are entitled to it. With what you give to your children and others each day, you more than earn the right to take good care of yourself. This time with your kids is very special and you should be able to enjoy it fully. You also deserve to tend to any problems caused by all the changes that come with being a mother.

Further, taking care of yourself is not selfish—it's good for others too. It's what you need to do in order to be at your best with your kids and still have some energy left over for your relationship with your partner. Just like in an airplane, you have to put on your own oxygen mask before you can help anyone else with theirs. A nurtured mother is the foundation of a healthy family.

Again and again, we see a minor miracle when a woman makes some simple changes in such things as what she eats, the way she thinks about stress, or how she talks with her partner. It's not complicated or esoteric. In the chapters that follow, we'll show you easy ways that work together and add up over time to nurture your body, mind, and important relationships.

HOW YOUR CUPBOARD CAN BECOME BARE

The first step is to understand exactly how raising a family has affected you personally. Once you've identified what's been happening for you, you've got a foundation for using the tools provided in the rest of the book.

Growing Demands on You

As demanding as parenthood has been for your mate, it has likely had even more impact on you. For starters, if you gave birth, you had the extraordinary task of building the most complex organ the body ever grows, using up to 80,000 extra calories to make your baby. If any nutrients were missing in the foods you ate, they were extracted from you and given to your child. When your baby was born, your placenta—which was a huge hormone factory during pregnancy—was dropped into the doctor's bucket, and within days after childbirth, your estrogen and progesterone fell to a fraction of their previous levels, gyrating the hormones that regulate everything from your mood when you wake up to how well you sleep at night.

If you breastfeed (about half of all mothers do—and we generally recommend it, for its benefits to both you and your child), each day you burn up an extra 450–500 calories: like running four to five miles a day. Breast milk is rich in nutrients such as essential fatty acids, which are vital for your baby, but you need these, too, for a healthy body and positive mood. If you are not eating enough of these nutrients in your regular diet, and few moms with infants seem to have the time, your bodily reserves are drained every time you nurse.

Plus, as one mother put it, *Real labor begins after birth.* Each day, for twenty-plus years, you'll do several hundred specific child-rearing or housework tasks, from reading *Winnie-the-Pooh* to doing the dishes, and you probably go to bed wishing that somehow you could have done more. The more committed you are to being sensitive and responsive to your child, the more work there is. One mother told Rick: *The biggest change was my sense that I had to always be present for and attentive to someone else, that I could never let down. I feel I am on call all the time.*

Besides being time-consuming, the work of mothers is uniquely stressful; the comedian Martin Mull once joked, *Having a family is like having a bowling alley installed in your brain.* Your body has been on a roller coaster from the first changes of pregnancy to childbirth, nursing, weaning, and the hormonal effects of chronic stress. Breastfeeding rarely proceeds without one troublesome hitch or another, especially in the beginning. You're constantly interrupted and pulled in a dozen different directions, you feel responsible for everything, things keep changing, worries gnaw at your mind, and something upsetting happens several times each day. Any wobble with your children wears on you further: You are probably the one, not your partner, who stumbles down the hall at night to tend to a baby with an ear infection, deals with childcare hassles, settles most squabbles between siblings, or worries about how to handle a preschooler's tantrums. As a result, mothers consistently report more stress than fathers, or women not raising children—especially if a child has any special needs, like colic, an illness, a disability, or a challenging temperament. And of course, the more kids, the more work and stress.

Adding to your stresses, you could be juggling home and work. Over half of all mothers today will return to work before their baby's first birthday—yet doing so while raising an infant increases their risk of health problems, especially if they're already stretched, such as by being a single parent. Toss in a steady stream of texts, emails, phone calls, and interruptions, and it can feel like your nervous system never gets a chance to settle down.

A Thin Soup of Resources

Meeting the growing demands that come with raising children requires increased resources. We're sure that one sort of resource has increased since you had children: the emotional fulfillment of being a mother. But otherwise, have your resources grown since your baby was born? Probably not. We're not talking about money here, but things like a good night's sleep and healthy foods and strong support from your partner and others. For instance, the typical mother of a young child gets about 6½ hours of sleep per day rather than the 8 or more hours most adults need—losing over 500 hours of sleep *per year*—plus she rarely gets a chance to sleep as deeply as she needs to. This diminishes the neurotransmitters her brain needs to regulate her mood and other physiological functions.

You're probably not eating all that well, either: Many mothers report skipping meals or eating irregularly. It's hard to find time to exercise with little ones around. And whether you're going off to the workplace or staying home, when you've got a young family, pleasures fall away, old friends drop out of your life, and you never seem to have any real time for yourself. Even if you're ill, you usually get little chance to rest. One mother told Jan this story: *I was reading a nursery rhyme to Julie, the one about Mother Hubbard, and I had to sigh because that's how I was starting to feel: My "cupboard" is constantly emptied while little gets put on the shelves.*

Has your partner jumped in to fill this vacuum? Maybe. Some dads are great: Skillful with the kids and committed to parenthood, they do their fair share around the house and are sympathetic and supportive. But let's face it: Many are not. Studies have found that the average mom works about 20 hours more per week, altogether, than does her partner, regardless of whether she's drawing a paycheck. You probably also handle more of the high-stress tasks, like dressing a resistant two-year-old, plus you likely carry more of the "executive responsibility" for the family by being the one who worries, plans, and problem-solves. And if you're raising your children essentially alone, as do one in five mothers, you're getting little to no help from a partner at all.

Even if your partner is a strong teammate, the arrival of children commonly leads to a dramatic decrease in positive interactions and relationship satisfaction—especially for mothers. There is so little time or energy for conversation, fun, or affection that there's a good chance your relationship no longer recharges your batteries or offers a safe haven. As one mother commented to Rick: *My husband and I work together well in terms of taking care of the kids and the house. But I don't know where he and I are as a couple apart from the kids and the house. I feel lonely inside my own marriage.* It's no wonder that couples with children report less satisfaction with their relationship than couples without kids.

Children are meant to be raised within a strong community, but compared to the times in which most of us grew up, relatives live farther away, neighbors are less neighborly, there are fewer kids nearby, and the average adult is affiliated with just one community group as compared to five in our parents' day. Compounding the problem, fathers have not entered the world of family to the extent that mothers have gone into the world of work, leaving a kind of vacuum, so there is less of the glue that once held neighborhoods together. As a result of all these factors, you're likely to have much less of the social support that could have provided practical help, lowered your stress, and buttressed your health.

In short, things have *really* changed, both in your own life since becoming a parent and in the culture since you were a child yourself, and chances are you simply aren't getting the kind of full support you need.

Vulnerable Spots in Your Armor of Resilience

In a perfect world, you could cope with all the demands on you combined with scarce resources by being some kind of Supermom. Yet that's not real. Each of us has some vulnerabilities that lower our resilience, the way a wound on a finger creates an opening for bacteria. Like a small cut that makes little difference until you do the dishes, often our vulnerabilities don't matter much before children arrive. But then these vulnerabilities worsen the effects of the demands upon you; for instance, an immune system weakened by chronic stress is less able to defend you against the germs brought home from preschool. And vulnerabilities also worsen the impacts of scant resources. For example, if you are even a little anemic when you enter motherhood—as up to 40 percent of women are—your nutritional reserves will be further eroded by the typical, low-iron diet of a mother.

Please see if any of these vulnerabilities, common among mothers, apply to you:

- **Having children at an older age:** In the last three decades, the birth rate of women over 30 has increased by about one-quarter, and the rate of first births for women over 35 has nearly doubled. It's just a fact: Older mothers are typically less able to weather a pregnancy, are more prone to fatigue and illness once children arrive, and have less time to restore a hormonal equilibrium before menopause.
- **Nutritional deficiencies:** About nine mothers in ten have not consumed the US government recommended amounts of minerals and vitamins before conceiving their first child. Nutritional deficiencies are cumulative, and since about a third of all pregnancies are unplanned, there's often little time to remedy

them before the demands of bearing and rearing a child gather a full head of steam. And even if you start taking supplements, it often takes months or years to restore healthy levels of nutrients in your body.

- **Genetic predisposition:** Your relatives may have had illnesses of the endocrine system, obstetric complications, or other conditions that raise your risk for similar issues.
- **Prior health problems:** Women are more likely than men to enter parenthood with preexisting gastrointestinal, hormonal, or autoimmune conditions.
- **Postpartum depression (PPD):** At least one mother in eight will have an episode of PPD, which can increase her risk for hormonal or mood-related problems a year or two later. And if you suffered from postpartum depression after your first baby, your chance triples of having PPD again with another child.
- **General history of depressed mood:** Some women have a tendency toward depression, and this can be intensified by the hormonal fluctuations of motherhood.
- **Temperament:** Raising kids is likely to be more stressful if a mother has a high need for control or orderliness, or if she tends to be anxious or irritable.

> *Improvements of the nutritional status of American women of childbearing age should be a national priority.*
>
> Gladys Block, PhD, and Barbara Adams, PhD

Some unique blend of vulnerabilities affects every mother. In the chapters that follow, we'll be teaching you how to shore up these vulnerabilities and increase your resilience so you're able to cope better with the increased demands upon you.

Swimming Upstream

Let's step back for a minute and look at how we got here. During more than 99 percent of the time that humans (or our close ancestors) have lived on this planet, mothers raised their families in small groups of hunter-gatherers. If you had been among them, your life would have moved at the speed of a walk while you provided for your needs and fulfilled your ambitions with a child on your hip or nearby. You would have eaten fresh and organic foods saturated in micronutrients and breathed air and drunk water free of artificial chemicals. Most important of all, you would have spent much of your day with other mothers, surrounded by a supportive community of relatives, friends, and neighbors—not alone or staring at a screen to make some kind of contact. These are the conditions to which your body and mind are adapted for raising children.

Unfortunately, while the essential activities of mothering—pregnancy, childbirth, breastfeeding, worrying and planning and loving with all your heart—have not altered one bit, our world has changed profoundly, and evolution hasn't had time to catch up. You and we are genetically identical to the first anatomically modern humans of 300,000 years ago, and nearly identical to our earliest tool-making ancestors, who lived over two million years ago. Nonetheless, at odds with this basic genetic blueprint, most mothers today must rush about stressfully, constantly juggling and multitasking. Few modern jobs can be done with young children around, so working means spending much of the day separated from your kids—and the stresses of the unnatural schedule and pace they must then handle affect them in ways that naturally spill over onto you. Compared to our ancestors, most of us eat much fewer vegetables and whole foods, and much more white flour, sugar, and highly processed foods, and we can't help absorbing some of the billions of pounds of toxins released into the environment each year, which even leave traces in breast milk. The so-called village it takes to raise a child usually looks more like a ghost town, so you have to rely more on your mate than did mothers in times past—but he, too, is strained by the unprecedented busyness and intensity of modern life.

If you feel like you're swimming upstream, it's because raising children was not meant to be this way. Many of the problems that seem purely personal or marital actually start on the other side of your front door.

Of course, the world is not going to change back to the time of the hunter-gatherers (and we'd miss refrigerators and smartphones too much if it did!). And those times certainly had their own difficulties, such as famine and disease. But, like every mother, you can't help but feel the impact of the whirlwind we're all living in. Just how you're affected is as individual as a baby's footprint. Some mothers are fortunate to have low demands upon them, substantial resources, and low vulnerabilities (see Figure 1). All too often, however, the demands are high, resources are low, and resilience gets worn down: A mother's "cupboard" gets emptied out and shaken, and it's an uphill struggle to get anything back in. No wonder that, over time, some signs of wear begin to show (see Figure 2).

Let's take a look now at how having kids affected the body, mind, or marriage of three different mothers—plus what they did to make things better.

Figure 1: Motherhood As It Should Be

CAUSES	*CONSEQUENCES*		
Workload and Stress	**Psychological**	**Physical**	**Relationships**
LOW TO MODERATE	Sense of coping	Energy	Good communication
Resources	Positive emotions	Full supply of nutrients	Teamwork
HIGH	Optimism	Balanced systems	Intimacy
Vulnerabilities	Normal mood	Health	Community
LOW			

Figure 2: Motherhood As It Often Is

CAUSES
Workload and Stress
HIGH
Resources
LOW
Vulnerabilities
HIGH

CONSEQUENCES		
Psychological	**Physical**	**Relationships**
Feeling overwhelmed	Fatigue	Poor communication
Negative emotions	Drained nutrients	Tension, conflict
Pessimism	Disturbed systems	Coldness, divorce
Depressed mood	Illness	Isolation

THE EFFECTS ON A MOTHER'S BODY

A year after Judy's* second child was born, she returned to Ricki's office for a routine follow-up visit. Judy was 43, dark-haired, slender, and edgy, with a no-nonsense gaze, and she worked full-time as a bookkeeper for a large trucking company. Her husband had moved out midway through her pregnancy, saying that he did not want another child. Ricki wondered if her ex-husband was giving her any help. Judy frowned: *Him? He takes Amanda to the park. When he feels like it.* But she smiled proudly when she added that Amanda and her older child, Matt, were doing fine, and the tough mask that got her through each day dropped away for a moment, revealing a tender warmheartedness.

Ricki asked what she was eating these days, and Judy snorted. *Who has time to cook? I've got friends without kids, and they tell me they're so busy. I just laugh because they have no idea what "busy" really is. I usually grab a bagel for breakfast, have a salad for lunch, and pick up some pizza or Chinese take-out for dinner.* She smiled. *Besides, it keeps the pounds off.*

When Ricki began going through a checklist of physical symptoms, Judy waved her hand: *Don't bother, I'm just on edge. I wake up*

* Identifying details have been altered in the examples given, which are sometimes composites of several mothers.

in the middle of the night and can't get back to sleep. Little things piss me off like never before, and I'm forgetting things I should know. She paused and straightened her shoulders. *I'm only tired. I feel like I'm running on fumes. Still, I'm kind of mad at myself for not doing a better job.*

But Ricki was concerned that there was more to Judy's case than simple fatigue. In addition to the high stresses of being a single mom raising two young children, Judy had several vulnerabilities: Her second child was born when she was 42, she had had gestational diabetes, and she had a family history of thyroid problems.

Therefore, Ricki ran several tests, and they revealed that Judy's blood sugars were elevated, while her thyroid levels were at the bottom of the normal range; Judy had also described some of the symptoms of insufficient thyroid, including cold hands and feet, fatigue, and hair loss. Meanwhile, Ricki had referred Judy to Jan for a nutritional evaluation. Just from hearing about her food habits, Jan could tell that Judy was not getting enough protein. Additionally, laboratory testing revealed that Judy had insufficient vitamin B6, which is critical for hormone balance and the production of serotonin, a neurotransmitter that helps regulate mood and digestion. Also, Judy was low on magnesium, which is essential for sleep, as well as taurine, an amino acid that helps a person feel both energized and relaxed.

Working together, Jan and Ricki helped Judy to:

- Lower her blood sugar levels through a low-sugar, low-carbohydrate diet.
- Restore balance to her hormones by taking a low dose of a natural thyroid medication.
- Increase her intake of protein, vitamins, minerals, and amino acids by eating in a healthier way. Jan gave Judy some tips on how to prepare quick yet nutritious meals (see chapter 4). In particular, Judy made sure to eat a lot of green leafy vegetables,

which are full of B-vitamins. She also started eating more seeds and beans for magnesium, and more meats (such as fish) for protein and taurine.

- Improve her nutrition further by taking a multivitamin/mineral supplement—as well as specific supplements for vitamin B6, magnesium, and taurine—since it is difficult to remedy nutritional deficiencies rapidly through diet alone.

It made Judy feel immediately better to realize that her low energy, poor memory, and irritability had been due in large part to physical causes, so they no longer seemed like a personal failing. And within a few weeks, her interventions dramatically improved her sleep and energy level, and helped her feel less tense and prickly at work and with her kids. In her final appointment, Judy smiled when she told Jan, *Now when I push my gas pedal, it feels like I've got something in the tank.*

Recognizing Depletion

As with many mothers who seem to have purely psychological concerns—such as irritability, poor memory, or a blue mood—there was, in fact, something awry with Judy's *body*. If there's one lesson that we've learned from working with several thousand mothers, it's the degree to which motherhood affects women physically. For example, the body of a woman generally reacts more intensely to stress than a man's does, and, like most mothers, you are probably living with more ongoing stress than anyone's body is meant to handle. It's important to realize that chronic stress is more than an unpleasant experience. It relentlessly disturbs many of your body's systems:

- **Gastrointestinal system**, by causing your mouth to produce less saliva, your stomach to secrete fewer digestive acids, and your small intestine to slow its contractions, which impairs nutrient absorption and can lead to irritable bowel syndrome and other digestive dysfunctions.

- **Nervous system**, by releasing certain neurotransmitters and hormones while suppressing others, leading to depressed mood and poorer concentration and memory.
- **Endocrine system**, by increasing such hormones (or related substances) as adrenaline and cortisol, and by lowering insulin, estrogen, progesterone, and DHEA, thereby raising the risk for type 2 diabetes, a poor response to stress, and other hormonal conditions.
- **Immune system**, by both weakening it and making it overreactive, leading to an increase in viral infections and autoimmune diseases.

It all adds up over time. You're pouring out more and handling more stresses, but taking less in. It's no wonder if you feel used up, emptied out—in a word, *depleted.* Besides being a psychological experience, your body could be getting depleted as well, which means that its vital nutrients are becoming drained and its key systems are getting dysregulated. Researchers have found signs of depletion in mothers from both middle-class American populations and low-income countries. Nonetheless, since the research on women's health has lagged far behind that of men, the long-term health effects of motherhood have not been well studied. Our analysis of depletion is a working hypothesis, based on existing data and our clinical experience, that we hope will be investigated further in future research.

Depletion is bad enough in its own right, but its effects today can also become causes of depletion tomorrow. For instance, as your mood sinks, it becomes harder to take steps to replenish yourself, like getting out of the house for some exercise. That's why it's important to take steps early on to prevent depletion in the first place: *The foundation of being a happy, healthy mom is nurturing your body.*

The demands on you may be greatest during your baby's first year, but it often takes a couple of years for the deepest reserves within your body to run dry. Therefore, we usually see the worst slump of depletion two or three years after the first child is born, or sometimes a year or so after a second child comes along. In general, things tend to get better by the time children are in grade school. Nonetheless, some mothers—typically those who are most stressed and least supported—continue to be depleted.

Of course, depletion is not the only health problem a mother might face: You could have a medical condition unrelated to raising children or one linked to motherhood—such as an injury suffered during childbirth—but not due to depletion. Nonetheless, any health issues become stresses that foster depletion, and depletion can worsen other bodily problems.

It should come as no surprise, then, that raising a family is associated with generally poorer health in a woman, especially as the number of her pregnancies increases. More specifically, some studies have shown or suggested that motherhood can raise a woman's risk for:

- fatigue
- nutritional deficits
- diabetes
- gallbladder disease
- a higher overall mortality rate
- cardiovascular disease
- hormonal problems
- kidney disease
- some kinds of cancer

The good news is that these are risks, not realities. You can lower them tremendously by preventing depletion in the first place, or by replenishing yourself if you've become depleted, using the strategies in the chapters that follow.

Depleted Mother Syndrome

Many mothers feel unnecessarily guilty about feeling worn out or blue, and many fathers do not really understand the full impact of motherhood. Some people might think that a mother "just has to snap out of it."

Well, if her body is seriously depleted, she can't just snap out of it! There is something physically wrong. We think she has a clinical condition that we term depleted mother syndrome (DMS). Like other syndromes such as premenstrual syndrome (PMS) or chronic fatigue syndrome (CFS), DMS can:

- Appear in a variety of forms.
- Be caused by different combinations of factors, depending on the person.
- Take a course over time that varies from mother to mother.
- Have symptoms that are ailments in their own right, such as depression.
- Respond to more than one kind of treatment.

How do you know if you have DMS? The gold standard, described in Appendix A, is medical lab testing of your nutrient levels, plus consideration by a doctor of any signs of disturbed systems. Meanwhile, you can use the checklists at the end of this chapter to get a sense of your risk of being depleted; the greater your risk, the more vital it is to try to lower the demands upon you and increase your resources.

If you are indeed depleted, you are far from alone. Based on our clinical experience, we estimate that at least one mother in ten will go through a period of measurable depletion. If you belong to a group of women with higher risks—such as childbirth past age 30, closely spaced pregnancies, prior health problems, single parenthood, or poverty—your chance of developing DMS will be higher.

Motherhood is not a medical issue, but depletion is. Every year, it impacts millions of American women and their family members, and it probably leads to billions of dollars in health care expenses and lost productivity. Since the physical, psychological, or interpersonal problems of mothers often originate in one place—depletion—understanding them as a syndrome enables diagnosis, prevention, and care to be directed at their root cause.

THE EFFECTS ON A MOTHER'S MIND

> *Evidence is accumulating that being a mother may be the most important source of stress in women's lives.*
>
> Rosalind C. Barnett, PhD,
> and Grace K. Baruch, PhD

Ann was 27, dark-haired, with a warm smile. She came to see Rick for ideas about her strong-willed, highly active, 18-month-old daughter. Ann had taken time off from her job managing a travel agency to stay home with Katie, who'd been adopted at birth. Her husband, Peter, worked long days and traveled frequently as a supervisor in a commercial construction company. At night, Katie still woke up several times and would cry for hours until someone picked her up. Peter said he needed to leave early in the morning to get to work, so Ann had to get up during the night, over and over.

Ann was embarrassed by Katie's intensity and frequent tantrums, and thought it had to be her fault that her daughter was acting that way, so she avoided getting together with other moms. Childcare was expensive, plus Ann felt "lazy" using it. As a result, she spent most of the day alone with her daughter. She rarely had a moment for herself, and she was constantly anxious about what Katie was going to get into next. Peter was helpful with Katie, but he was gone so much of the time. When he was around, Ann felt uncomfortable saying outright how close to the edge she occasionally got, and he did not pick up on her hints.

She tried so hard to be loving and patient with Katie. But sometimes she felt overwhelmed with anger when her daughter was really defiant, *like a switch flips and I become another person,* and it was all she could do not to hit her. Then she felt ashamed of her reactions and was full of self-recrimination.

Ann had not slept well for over a year, either just waiting for Katie to wake up the next time, or restless with guilt and worry. She told Rick that she felt worn out, sad, or irritable most of the time, and her face was lined and weary.

Once all this had been laid out on the table, Rick told her that many other mothers had similar feelings. They discussed the harsh logic of Ann's situation: Even without the biological demands of pregnancy or nursing, sleep deprivation plus high stress had combined with low support to make her feel irritable and angry, anxious, guilty and inadequate, and depressed. Just hearing that her reactions were not abnormal, and that there were reasons for them, felt calming and hopeful to Ann.

Storms of Anger

Ann felt most concerned about the "amazing anger" that came over her. Rick pointed out that many parts of raising a child would irritate anyone but a saint, such as trying to change a stinky diaper while your toddler kicks and thrashes. Because they feel bad about getting mad at their kid, mothers tend to push these angry feelings down. Then they fester and grow, sometimes erupting. It's a rare parent who has never lost it with a child. The fact that Ann was worried about raging at Katie showed that she knew she shouldn't hit her daughter in anger.

Rick asked how she had been brought up, since every parent is affected by experiences from childhood—like "ghosts in the nursery," in the memorable phrase of Professor Selma Fraiberg. Ann had grown up in a strict and emotionally cool home. She had become very self-critical, and each struggle with Katie seemed like more proof that she was not a good person.

Fears and Worries

Ann was like so many mothers who have increased feelings of anxiety after having children. Not just the reasonable concerns everyone has—*Why is he crying? What was that crash?*—but a nagging sense of apprehension, worry, or fear. This generalized anxiety was as far as it went for Ann, but some mothers also experience one or more acute conditions:

- The stresses of mothering can lead to panic attacks, which are sudden, overwhelming states of fear and physical discomfort.
- Because many aspects of parenting are beyond anyone's control—such as a child's temperament—a mother may become preoccupied with irrational worries, or compulsive about things she *can* control, like laying out clothes or washing her hands.
- If her child has major health problems or is seriously injured, she could suffer the symptoms of acute stress disorder at the time—such as things seeming unreal, feeling numbed, intrusive thoughts or images, or heightened reactivity—or post-traumatic stress disorder (PTSD) at a later point.

Feeling Guilty or Inadequate

Ann and Rick also talked about how motherhood was a strange combination of feeling wonderful and worthless. You're the most important person in the world to your children and half of the all-American equation of "motherhood and apple pie." On the other hand, you feel terrible that you can't figure out why the baby is crying or like an idiot trying to get a toddler to eat cooked carrots. Others—including strangers in the supermarket—point out how you could do a better job. During the time you're home with children, you lose a source of pride and status through accomplishments at work.

The way you think about all this makes a big difference in how you feel. In Ann's mind, any little error was highlighted. Yet the many good things she did each day with her daughter were brushed aside. No wonder that, like many women, her sense of worth declined since becoming a mother.

Disturbed Mood

These knocks against self-esteem are just one of the many conditions faced by mothers that are known to cause depression. The rest include sleep deprivation, overwork, stress, changes in physical appearance, ongoing issues with children (such as problems with childcare, a health problem, or a challenging temperament), health concerns, marital conflict, and social isolation—all of which applied to Ann, so it wasn't surprising that she had gotten depressed.

While raising children, you've got about a 50-50 chance of going through a period of depressed mood—lasting at least several weeks, and potentially a year or more—when you feel sad, discouraged, or emotionally numb much of the time. You may experience less interest or pleasure in activities that used to be enjoyable, and even the joys of raising a child can feel blanketed by a gloomy cloud. Relatively small things could seem like big problems, and it's much easier to get irritated or frustrated. You may have a loss of appetite, increase in fatigue, or disturbance in sleep. Besides being a waking nightmare for you, depression wears more on a marriage than any other health problem.

Getting the Weight Off Your Mind

Ann chose to work with Rick for a few months. During that time, she took steps that we'll describe in detail in the next three chapters, such as:

- She started using cognitive techniques to argue back against overly self-critical thinking, such as listing several accurate and positive thoughts to refute a distorted and negative one. And by reflecting on her childhood, she was able to sort out sensible reactions to here-and-now situations from unreasonable responses that were amplified by the past. Because she started feeling less like a "bad mom," she enrolled Katie in a co-op preschool a few mornings each week, and her daughter really liked it. At the school, she met some other moms and became good friends with two of them.
- With her extra time, she began exercising again. In particular, she returned to activities that had once given her pleasure, including long bike rides.
- She now took little moments, that she would have previously ignored, to get some stress relief, such as taking a bath instead of her usual quick shower.
- Feeling more self-respect helped her tell Peter that it was only fair for him to get up more often in the night with Katie. She also read up on methods for parenting a spirited child and helping a child learn to sleep through the night. To her pleasant surprise, some of them actually worked.

These actions began showing results within the first weeks. Katie responded to Ann's changes in parenting style and became more cooperative. She was still packed with punch, but now her squabbles stayed mainly in bounds. Ann's nervous anticipation of the next disaster faded, and she began feeling better about herself as a mother—and person.

Within a few months, Ann reported less sadness and more vitality. Her growing connections with other moms improved her self-confidence as a mother, as studies have shown with other women. Also, they probably increased the effectiveness of her immune system, another research finding, which helped cut down on her colds.

She began looking like her original vibrant and athletic self. She had the normal ups and downs of anyone, but she wasn't depressed anymore. She and Rick wrapped up their work together, and he asked her to keep in touch. About a year later he was delighted to receive a card from her: On the cover was a lovely picture of the baby boy that she and her husband had just adopted. Rick called to see how she was doing. They were "nuts," she admitted, but there was a bounce and sense of confidence in her voice that said she and Peter and her two children were going to be fine. All the little steps she had taken for her well-being had paid off—just like your own steps will too.

THE EFFECTS ON A MOTHER'S MARRIAGE

Couples are affected in different ways by the arrival of children: Some weather the stresses and changes very well, while others are seriously strained—sometimes to the breaking point. The good news is that if there have been breakdowns in teamwork or intimacy, they can usually be repaired if one or ideally both partners makes a real effort to work on them, and chapters 6, 7, and 8 will show you how.

For example, Maria and Alex began seeing Rick when their two boys, Josh and Sam, were four and a half and two years old. Maria was 33 and had worked as an operating room nurse before staying home with their sons. Her hazel eyes were warm, and like many nurses, she had a meticulous, conscientious manner. Alex was a good deal older, 46, and they had met at the hospital where he continued to work as an orthopedic surgeon. He had curly dark hair shot with gray, weary brown eyes, and a measured, scholarly style of speaking.

In their first session, Maria said that Alex never got home when he said he would. He was OK with the boys but so strict that she felt she always had to intervene. He wouldn't think for himself about what they needed, so she had to keep telling him what to do, and it seemed that whenever she turned around, he had disappeared into his study to catch up on paperwork or emails.

Then she added that he gave her no support with the issues of raising a preschooler and a toddler. She was continually weighing "a million details" about the boys. Naturally, she wanted to talk things over with him. But when she finally got him to sit down, he usually interrupted her with some superficial quick fix or rolled his eyes like she was an idiot. She felt her concerns were well considered, and she was flabbergasted, hurt, and increasingly angry about him treating her like an incompetent orderly.

Alex's eyes were troubled when Maria finished, and he kept shaking his head. He finally said that she needed to "quit obsessing" about the kids. He put a high value on self-reliance and felt Maria was too indecisive and needy. *She was the best nurse I ever had, so I do not understand why she cannot simply solve these child-management problems on her own.* He thought she needed to exercise better self-control and not use him as a lightning rod when it was the boys she was actually upset with. Besides, when he wanted to talk about something from work, *You can tell she's thinking about something else.*

Then he spoke even more stiffly, but the embarrassment and hurt leaked through: *Maria nurses Sam to sleep in the boys' bedroom and usually falls asleep there herself. I think our personal relationship would be improved if we arranged to end up in the same bed. I must tell you that we have not had intimate relations in a year.*

Feeling Let Down

When Alex finished, the air was heavy with disappointment. Like many parents, each of them had reasons to feel let down by the other. Maria wanted a partnership of the heart in the greatest undertaking of her life. Instead, she felt fended off, patronized, and turned into a "management problem."

Alex, however, felt he was holding up his end of what in some quarters had been a traditional bargain—Dad makes a living and Mom runs the household—so why couldn't Maria? From his own experience as a parent, Rick shared that as a new father he'd had to change the way he looked at things: Having children means that your partner is understandably and unavoidably dependent on *you* (which, by the way, could be uncomfortable and scary for her), you are no longer a free agent, and you have to be aware of how your actions affect her. Like every father, Alex also needed to recognize that he bore some responsibility for his wife's fatigue and concerns, since she was raising *his* children, and therefore he needed to give her some help with them.

Additionally, the typical disturbance in a couple's erotic relationship after children had affected Maria and Alex. There was little of the foundation of positive feelings, conversation, and nonsexual touch that Maria needed in order to feel comfortable making love. Even if these had been present, the deep fatigue, hormonal disruption of libido, feeling pulled on all day, and logistical difficulties experienced by all new parents would still have complicated their sex life.

If you are nodding your head in recognition, you might be thinking that your partner should be willing to set aside some of his personal needs for a year or two, just like you have. But the crux for a man usually isn't the lack of sex per se, but the sense that he does not seem to matter enough to his partner to care about him as a lover. Like many men, Alex felt there was as little room for him in Maria's heart as there was in her bed.

Eight Times as Many Arguments

Alex and Maria saw Rick off and on for about a year. A few weeks after their first session, in response to Alex's ongoing complaints about the lack of sex, Maria shot back: *If I can't trust you to get home on time, if I can't trust you not to be too hard on the boys, and if I can't trust you to listen to me when I'm upset, why would I trust you in bed?*

Alex hemmed and hawed. Rick asked him how he'd feel about a member of his operating team who was as shaky about his work commitments as Alex was at home. After a pained silence, Alex said gruffly, *I can see the point.*

Kids bring an intense need for teamwork, but a mother and father often disagree about childrearing or how to share the load fairly. As a result, researchers have found that the average couple has eight times as many arguments after children arrive—a major reason why two couples in three report a sharp drop in satisfaction with their relationship once they become parents. Struggles with your partner over child-rearing are intensely distressing and can lead to psychological problems. And besides feeling awful, these quarrels wear on your health, in part by increasing your blood pressure and weakening your immune system.

Issues related to parenting last as long as kids do. If they are not resolved, the same quarrels happen again and again, and they become increasingly charged. Over time, positions harden, and each person becomes more defended. Then the other one figures they had better bring the heavy artillery—which leads to even more defensiveness. Mistrust grows in vicious cycles. The fights get even worse. You once walked down the aisle thinking you could place your life in this man's hands. Now you could find yourself eyeing him as an unreliable character who must be cajoled or corralled into reasonable and helpful behavior. And, sometimes, that may be how he's looking at you too.

A Chilly Distance

Each time either parent feels misunderstood, let down, or angry cuts thread by thread at the emotional cords binding them together. A few months into therapy, Maria described an episode that had occurred when Josh was just two months old. At that time she felt deeply fatigued and vulnerable. Alex thought it would be good for their relationship if they went out, and he insisted they leave their son with a sitter and attend an outdoor concert with people from work. She protested but felt too worn out to put up much resistance. They ended up going, despite the fact that it was a cold and windy day. She worried about her baby the whole time, and she felt chilled to the bone. She was stunned, saddened, and outraged that her husband was so out of touch with how she was feeling. As she put it four years later, *I took a big step back from him that night, and haven't come fully forward since then.*

Some couples manage to mend these tears in the fabric of their marriage and preserve a strong and loving friendship. But in many cases, a chill fills the air at a time when it could have been so sweet to raise a child together. Their relationship shrinks to a size that feels safe: perhaps a bland, distant partnership for raising children and little else. For example, one mother said to Rick: *My husband tried to be helpful. But I wasn't giving him much attention, I was irritable all the time, and after a while he just gave up and withdrew. I was so devoted to my children that it seemed selfish of him to want to take my time away from them. Eventually, once I stopped nursing and started getting more sleep, I began to feel like my old self again. But by then, my husband had been withdrawn for so long it had become a kind of permanent state. Our marriage has never been the same.*

> *For many couples, the cascade toward divorce begins with the first decline in the wife's marital satisfaction after the arrival of the first baby.*
>
> Alyson Fearnley Shapiro, PhD, John M. Gottman, PhD, and Sybil Carrere, PhD

For Maria and Alex, things hit bottom about three months into the therapy. Maria said, *I don't think he loves me anymore. When you love somebody, when you really like them, you act a certain way. He doesn't act that way and I think the reason is simple.* She paused and asked him point blank: *Do you still love me?* Alex stared at his feet and chose his words carefully: *I think you are a terrific mother and we have many interests and values in common.* He went on like this until she interrupted him, her voice rising: *But do you* love *me?* There was a long pause before he looked her in the eye and said, *I hope so. But I'm not sure anymore.* Maria just stared at him. He finally spoke up, getting upset for the first time in their sessions: *Well, what about you? Are you interested in me—as a person, beyond the fact that I'm the father of your sons?* She answered, *There was a long time when I was actively not interested in you, basically paying you back for how you treated me. That's gotten better since coming here. I'm up to neutral. But I'm not yet up to real positive.*

A family therapist hears many loud and angry things. But the worst one of all is the quiet admission between two parents, said one way or another: *I don't love you anymore.* You're aware of their children, and what's at stake. His chair and hers are only a few feet apart. But they peer at each other as if across a great divide, each one trying to see the person they once loved, trying to find the love that used to flow so generously.

Maria and Alex looked over the edge of the abyss and did not like what they saw: separate households, the impact on their boys, less time with their sons, financial upheaval, trying to find a new partner. They realized that the real stakes when they fought were not the overt issues on the table—whatever those happened to be that day—but the future of their marriage. This was a turning point, and they got it, viscerally, that they had better repair their relationship faster than they were tearing it up.

Reknitting a Marriage

Over the course of a year, Maria and Alex used many of the tools and skills that you'll find in chapters 6, 7, and 8. They each made a unilateral commitment for several months to doing what they could do *personally* to have their relationship go better, independent of what the other person did. They did their best to live by the "80-20" rule: Put 80 percent of your attention on the corrections you can make and 20 percent on what your partner can do better.

With this commitment as a foundation, they established basic ground rules for civility, such as not fighting in front of the children, no name-calling, and no dragging the kids into their arguments. Alex tried to "lead with empathy" when Maria was worried or upset, rather than try to solve her problem, and Maria paid closer attention to Alex's stories about work. As a result, they began understanding each other better. Alex saw that Maria's focus on their sons was normal and not a personal rejection, and she realized that he had lost a wife in some ways while not gaining the moment-to-moment fulfillment she had with the children.

They worked on translating their complaints about the past into specific requests for the future. They learned how to negotiate about parenting, schedules, and the way they spoke to each other. For instance, Alex started controlling his temper with the boys and Maria stopped micromanaging him. Alex agreed to come home by six on Tuesdays and Thursdays and take care of the boys the rest of the evening. Besides giving Maria a couple nights off, he became immediately more understanding about what it was like to spend many hours alone with young children.

It was uncomfortable at first, but they started touching each other again with little pats and hugs. Rather than being passively resentful, Alex began gently rousing Maria after she put Sam to sleep. They started sleeping in the same bed. After a few months, they broke the ice and made love again. They realized that sex wasn't going to be as spontaneous as it used to be, and they came to an understanding that they would try to make love once a week or so.

Maria asked Alex if he could please try to be less stuffy. Bit by bit, he started talking with her more openly, awkwardly at first but growing increasingly at ease with it. Just the fact that he was making an effort warmed Maria's heart to him, and her greater friendliness in turn evoked in him more caring for her. Over time, the chill between them thawed, and the warm feelings that had drawn them together in the first place started to return. Six months after they began seriously working on their relationship, lying in bed together on a Saturday morning, Maria said three simple words to Alex that she had last spoken two years before: *I love you.* He was startled and became quiet. Then, when he spoke, his voice was firm: *I love you too.*

YOUR PATH TOWARD WELL-BEING, HEALTH, AND SUPPORT

Raising children is deeply fulfilling. Yet it's also intensely demanding. Compared to women who haven't had children, mothers are generally more stressed, more unhappy in their marriages, and more prone to illness. But if we've learned one thing in our personal lives and professional practices, it's that *none* of that distress or depletion is necessary! We outline the steps in the rest of this book, and they're fundamentally simple: Decrease the "bad"—the demands upon you—and increase the "good"—your resources and resilience. Everything works together. For example, research shows that greater support from your partner can boost your own physical and psychological health.

We know it's hard to take care of yourself when you've got a little one (or ones) on your hands. We've each been there ourselves and we see it all the time in our practices. But nurturing yourself *is* entirely possible, even with kids to manage and a household to run. In the chapters to come, you'll see how to get the stress relief, nutrition, health care, teamwork, and intimacy you need. Together, these methods will prevent depletion and build up your well-being, so that this wonderful time in your life is as good as it can possibly be. That's what being a happy, healthy mom is all about.

Key Risk Factors for Depletion

In order to see where your risks for depletion lie—and therefore where to focus your efforts—please check the boxes that apply to you. Wherever possible, chapters are indicated in which you will find help for that risk. And to get a sense of your overall risk for depletion, add up the number of boxes you marked. Five or fewer factors suggest low risk, six to fifteen factors suggest moderate risk, and sixteen or more factors suggest high risk.

HIGH DEMANDS UPON YOU

Physical

[ ] Have had two or more children

[ ] Less than 18 months spacing between children

[ ] Breastfed one or more children for longer than 18 months

[ ] Breastfed during pregnancy, or two children during the same period

[ ] Became pregnant and carried to term less than three months after weaning the previous child

[ ] Disturbed sleep over past three months, or averaged less than seven hours per day (Chapter 4)

Child-related

[ ] Currently caring for a child under age three

[ ] Care for a child eight or more hours a day

[ ] Child with challenging temperament (e.g., spirited, stubborn, aggressive, fearful)

[ ] Child with chronic physical or psychological problems

Associated factors

[ ] Unreliable or mediocre childcare (Chapter 9)

[ ] Substantial care of others besides children (e.g., ill spouse or parent)

[ ] Returned to work 20+ hours per week before baby was one year old (Chapter 9)

[ ] Currently working for pay 30+ hours per week or full-time student (Chapter 9)

LOW RESOURCES COMING TO YOU

Physical (Chapter 4)

[ ] During pregnancy(ies), ate less than three meals per day, or few fresh vegetables, or little protein

[ ] Since birth of first child, nutrition has been mediocre or poor

[ ] Little use of vitamin/mineral supplements

[ ] Little or no exercise

Psychological (Chapter 2)

[ ] Little time for breaks or personal enjoyments

[ ] Little use of stress relief techniques such as progressive relaxation or meditation

[ ] Have few personal enjoyments or pleasures

[ ] Little or no spiritual or religious orientation

Interpersonal

[ ] Single parent

[ ] Partner travels frequently (Chapters 6 and 7)

[ ] Low sense of teamwork or cooperation with partner (Chapters 6 and 7)

[ ] Partner does little child-rearing or housework during evenings or weekends (Chapters 6 and 7)

[ ] Low sense of emotional intimacy with a partner (Chapter 8)

[ ] Little affection or sexuality with a partner (Chapter 8)

[ ] Little tangible support from relatives

[ ] Little sense of connection with other mothers

[ ] Little sense of connection with community institutions supportive of families

PERSONAL VULNERABILITIES

Prior to pregnancy of first child

[ ] Extensive dieting or eating disorder (Chapter 4)
[ ] Generally mediocre or poor nutrition (Chapter 4)
[ ] Little use of vitamin/mineral supplements (Chapter 4)
[ ] Significant exposure to toxic chemicals (Chapter 4)
[ ] Hormone problems (e.g., thyroid disorder, diabetes, severe PMS) (Chapter 5)
[ ] Gastrointestinal problems (e.g., irritable bowel syndrome, digestive parasites, ulcer) (Chapter 5)
[ ] Immune system problems (e.g., severe allergies, asthma, arthritis, lupus) (Chapter 5)
[ ] Significant depression or anxiety (Chapters 3 and 5)
[ ] Family history of hormone, gastrointestinal, immune, or reproductive problems (Chapter 5)
[ ] Family history of psychological problems (Chapters 2 and 3)
[ ] Highly sensitive, anxious, or rigid temperament (Chapters 2 and 3)

During any pregnancy carried to term

[ ] Complications such as preeclampsia or toxemia
[ ] Serious obstetric complications

Since children

[ ] One or more children born when mother was 30+ years old
[ ] One or more episodes of postpartum depression (Chapters 3 and 5)
[ ] Regular use of tobacco (Chapter 4)
[ ] Alcohol abuse (e.g., needing to drink daily to cope, having more than 7 drinks per week) (Chapter 4)
[ ] Regular use of recreational drugs (Chapter 4)
[ ] Significantly overweight (Chapter 4)

PART TWO

Nurturing Your Mind

Whether it's middle-of-the-night feedings, daily battles with your toddler over wearing shoes, or a call from kindergarten to say that your daughter's taken a bad fall off the jungle gym, raising children, taken as a whole, will probably be the most stressful experience of your life. It can also bring on some of the most intensely painful feelings you've ever experienced, including sadness, anxiety, shame, and anger.

In chapter 2, you'll learn about strategies for coping with parental stress. Our goal is to give you a whole range of methods so that no matter how busy or frazzled you are, you'll have some tools to get you through. The idea is first to get immediate stress relief, and then—over the long term—to build up your psychological resilience: the capacity to cope with and recover quickly from your stresses.

Next, in chapter 3, we focus on the normal but difficult emotions that typically increase in the first years of parenthood, like sadness at the loss of a part of your old life before children, or irritation at your partner's casual assumption that it's mainly your job, not his, to manage your young child in a restaurant. We'll show you how to release these feelings and replace them with more positive ones.

Of course, addressing your inner experience—be it a general sense of stress or a specific emotion—will not itself change challenging circumstances such as problems with your childcare. But it can help you deal with them more effectively, or at least endure them more calmly. Similarly, a psychological intervention may not improve a health problem that's dragging you down, but the mind and body are interconnected, and upgrading your "software" can often improve your "hardware" as well; you'll find specific help for health in part 3. And in part 4, we'll cover a key source of stress relief: a supportive relationship with your partner.

CHAPTER TWO

Reducing Your Stress

Nobody likes being stressed, and it might seem like nothing can help. But it's important to remember that there is always *something* you can do to feel at least a little better. Right now, for instance, try shifting in your seat, loosening tight clothing, putting down your phone, or taking a full breath. It's a small thing, but it shows you *can* affect your own stress level.

You might feel some resistance to taking a moment to be kind to yourself, either within you or from the people around you. If this is true, you're certainly not alone. From childhood onward, girls and women are typically socialized to focus on the needs of others, and they can have a hard time taking care of their own. A mother's commitment to her children's welfare is usually so intense that it's naturally hard to pay attention to herself. We've heard mothers say things like *How can I take a bath or even a nap when my kids need me?* And sometimes other people can make you feel guilty for daring to try. A client of Rick's with a two-year-old plus a newborn was talking with her own mom about how tired she was. Her mother interrupted impatiently, *That is just mothering, you may as well get used to it,* and then changed the subject, as if she were passing down some unwritten rule of motherhood: *I suffered, and so should you.*

To us, this view is deeply wrong. Nurturing yourself is what *enables* you to be at your best for your children, day after day, year after year. One mother told us: *The times I have really blown it with my kids have all come when I was at the end of my rope. I remember moms with older kids telling me to take care of myself. I thought, "Yeah, sure," and kept on going full tilt. But they were right, and I wish I had realized that earlier.* Further, mothering is not a hobby you picked up for fun. You work hard for the sake of your children and family, and that *entitles* you to respect, care—and stress relief.

You Matter

Please consider these questions:

When you were growing up, how did your parents or others treat your needs and wants?

Currently, how do you treat your own needs and wants? Deep down, how much do you feel they matter? Deep down, how much do you feel that you *matter as a person altogether?*

In the "pie" of your typical day, how big is the slice that is lived just for you? If you felt like you mattered more as a person, how might that slice change?

Helmer: First and foremost, you are a wife and mother.
Nora: That I don't believe anymore. I believe that first and foremost I am an individual, just as much as you are.

Henrik Ibsen, *A Doll's House*

SHORT-TERM STRESS RELIEF

Even in the middle of the busiest day, there are lots of things you can do that will immediately lower your stress level and help you both feel better and create some space in which you can begin to figure out how to lower your stresses over the long term. Additionally, getting the needle on your personal stress meter out of the red zone stops the current wear and tear on your body, and it helps prevent your brain and hormones from getting so sensitized to stress that they overreact to it in the future.

That's why we recommend that you try to *feel good* as often as you can, at least several times each day. These experiences are more than enjoyable: They help protect your body against stress, improve problem-solving, and stop downward spirals. The occasional getaway for a weekend is great, but regular, daily, positive experiences will make much more difference for you in the long run.

Below, we've listed lots of ways to get your stress meter into the green. Many of these will take only a minute or so. While others take a little longer, you can do many of them while nursing, tending to children, doing housework, or driving. And of course we heartily encourage you to use whatever stress-reducing techniques you have discovered on your own as well. It's great simply to recognize that there are many, many little practical things you *can* do, no matter what your situation is, that will lower your stress. First aid for frazzled nerves is the first step toward a more stress-free you.

One-Minute Soothers

- Take four long, slow breaths, and as you exhale, imagine that a cloud of stress, worries, or troubles is leaving your life, and as you inhale, imagine that peace and love and wisdom are filling you up.

- Take your shoes off, rub the bottoms of your feet with your knuckles, and massage the joints and tips of your toes.
- Put your phone face-down or in another room for one minute and let your eyes rest on something real—your child's face, a tree outside, the sense of your own breath.
- Smell something nice, like an orange or your child's hair, or put on a dab of perfume.
- Roll your head around to loosen your neck.
- Splash water on your face.
- While standing, bend over to touch the floor, shake your arms loosely, and straighten up slowly as you take in a big breath.
- Look at something pretty.
- Knead your neck and shoulders.
- Nibble something good.
- Rub your eyes and the bones around them gently.
- Hug your child or partner for one whole minute.
- Stretch your mouth open as wide as you can, like a lion roaring, and then let your face relax.
- Remember a good joke.
- Repeat a favorite saying or prayer to yourself.

Five-Minute Soothers

- Make yourself a cup of tea.
- Lie down, close your eyes, and imagine a warm, golden balm settling over you, softening the edges of your feelings and gently carrying away any distress.
- Listen to your favorite music.
- Ask someone for a sincere compliment.
- Step outside and watch the play of sunlight dancing on leaves, or look up at the moon and the stars.
- Do a few minutes of stretching or yoga.

When you are a mother, you are never really alone in your thoughts. A mother always has to think twice, once for herself and once for her child.

Sophia Loren

Fifteen-Minute Soothers

- Take a long shower.
- Read a magazine.
- Go for a short walk and look for beauty.
- Arrange flowers in a vase.
- Cuddle up with your children or your partner.
- Call a friend for a quick chat.
- Be especially loving with someone instead of texting or messaging.
- Lie down for a brief nap.
- Meditate for fifteen minutes.
- Exercise, dance, stretch, or do yoga.

Thirty-Minute Soothers

- Read a good book.
- Take a bath—maybe with bubbles.
- Watch a TV show.
- Go for a walk.
- Treat yourself to a good nap.
- Trade a neck rub or foot massage with your partner.
- Do some art or a craft.
- Play a musical instrument.
- Call a friend and really talk.

One-Hour Soothers

- Go for a run, swim, or bike ride, even if you have to arrange special childcare to get this time to yourself.

- Get a manicure.
- Go out to lunch with your partner, a friend, or a good book.
- Visit your church or temple.
- Browse through a bookstore.
- Go for a walk in a park.
- Prepare a really nice meal just for yourself or treat yourself to a special lunch.

A Word on Technology Use and Stress

Technology has done many wonderful things for parents: It lets us arrange grocery pickups online, find encouragement and a sense of community when we feel alone, and simplify everyday logistics like scheduling. But it can also steal your sleep, feed constant comparisons, and distance you from your child or partner when they are missing your presence. All of that to say: *use technology, but don't let it use you*. If you can, try being off screens for the last hour before bed to support better sleep, and set a couple of small "phone-free" pockets during the day (mealtimes and bedtime are a great start). And if you notice that social media leaves you more anxious, down, or keyed up, consider a brief reset—even a day or a weekend away from it—and see how you feel.

LONG-TERM STRESS RELIEF

Immediate stress relief feels great, but it's also important to build up your psychological resilience for the long term. The essence is simple: First, *let go of the "bad,"* like tension, sadness, or troubling thoughts. Then, when you have released these burdens on your mind, you will have created a space in yourself in which to *take in the "good,"* such as positive experiences of happiness and self-worth. You can prevent or reduce depletion by the regular practice of these fundamental stress-reduction techniques. And over time, that practice will make a lasting difference in your own psychology and even your physiology, leading to improved mood and greater insight into yourself and other people.

You can let go of stress in each part of your inner world, including your body sensations, mental images, emotions, desires, and thoughts. Let's begin with the body.

> *The quickest way for a parent to get a child's attention is to sit down and look comfortable.*
>
> Lane Olinghouse

Relaxing Your Body

There are many ways to relax your body even in the middle of a busy day. You've already seen some in the previous section, and here are some additional ideas:

- A few times each day, try sweeping your attention through your body, noticing the places that are tight or uncomfortable, and consciously relaxing them. Key places to look for tension include your eyes, jaws and tongue, diaphragm (located just below the rib cage), and pelvic floor.
- After going to bed but before falling asleep, you can systematically relax the parts of your body. Just bring your awareness to each part—left foot, right foot, left ankle, etc., all the way up to your scalp—and let it relax.
- Breathing techniques are great ways to relax. Just take a big breath and let it out slowly. Try to breathe from your diaphragm by placing your hand on your stomach just below the arch of your rib cage and having each inhalation push your hand away from your backbone. Or inhale deeply and hold it

for a few seconds before exhaling gradually. Try not inhaling for a few seconds after you exhale. Perhaps imagine that your breath is going in and out of some tense part of your body; for example, you could get a sense that you are breathing into a tight neck or nervous stomach. Or try some techniques from yoga, such as inhaling through the nose and exhaling through the mouth; inhaling through your left nostril (closing the right one gently) and exhaling through the right nostril (closing the one on the left); taking several breaths by following a rhythmic count: inhale for five, hold for twenty, exhale for ten, and hold the exhalation for ten (adjust the pace of the count for your own comfort); or breathing rapidly and forcefully in and out of your nose for half a minute or more. "Box breathing" is also popular, in which you inhale for a count of 4, hold for 4, exhale for 4, and hold the exhalation for 4 . . . over and over again.

- When lying down, imagine being very heavy, so weighty that you are sinking down into the earth.
- Imagine that your hands are getting very warm, as if you're opening your hands toward a cheery fire or holding a cup of hot cocoa; this is especially helpful for going to sleep.
- Tense your arms or legs for a few seconds and then relax.

Resources for Letting Go

The Relaxation Response, by Herbert Benson

Focusing, by Eugene Gendlin

Being Peace, by Thich Nhat Hanh

The Relaxation and Stress Reduction Workbook, by Martha Davis, Mathew McKay, and Elizabeth Eshelman

Using Mental Imagery to Release Stress

Now that you've got more on your to-do list than ever, the internal running commentary inside your mind can drown out pretty much everything else, like the loudmouthed chair of a committee who won't let anyone else have the floor. But most of the brain itself is dedicated to nonverbal processes. That realm is a vital part of who you are, and by becoming more able to enter the fertile, wise world of images, daydreaming, and fantasy, you'll gain both stress relief and self-knowledge. Whenever you get tired of the yammering voice in the back of your head—maybe it just said, "What voice?"—you can try one of these suggestions:

- Recall or imagine a relaxing experience. Maybe you're on a tropical beach, feeling the warm sun and a gentle breeze playing on your skin, with the soft murmuring of happy people—perhaps your children—nearby. Or you could be walking across a mountain meadow, surrounded by wildflowers and the sound of babbling brooks, with the crisp smell of distant snow in the air. Try picking images of situations that are the opposite of the ones that are causing you stress. For example, if you feel like you're failing to solve a problem with your child, you might imagine successfully skiing down a challenging slope, or if you feel stuck in a sticky situation at work, imagine sailing freely under gorgeous skies.
- Visualize your body filled with colored liquid and little faucets at the tips of your fingers and toes. Open the taps and let the liquid drain out, taking with it all of the tension within you. Notice any remaining liquid, indicating stress that is not yet released, and encourage every bit of it to drain out of you.
- Imagine stresses or upsetting experiences flowing out of you each time you exhale, like a smoggy cloud exiting whenever

you blow out a breath. Or get a sense that you are standing in a warm and beautiful river, and that the water is cleansing you of stress, carrying it away and out to sea.

- If you've had an upsetting experience that you'd like to let go of, imagine putting it on a rocket and sending it to burn up in the sun, or on a big red balloon that disappears into the sky, or on a raft that floats down a river to the sea. If it's meaningful to you, you could imagine releasing it to whatever is spiritual for you.

Releasing Emotions

One of the challenges of motherhood is finding good ways to express your feelings. After all, you can hardly tell your toddler that you feel depressed or that his whining makes you want to scream. But emotion is like a river: When it's allowed to flow, it stays clean and clear, but when it's dammed up, it grows dank and smelly. Fortunately, there are two ways to release your feelings that do not require communicating directly: expressing them within your own mind and expressing them symbolically. (We'll discuss direct communication with your partner in chapters 6, 7, and 8.)

Expressing emotion within your own mind. The safest way to express emotion is to yourself, which doesn't reveal how you feel to anyone else. As a start, and as best you can, try to name your feelings to yourself. Normal emotions include joy, surprise, curiosity, love, peacefulness, sense of worth, triumph, religious exaltation, fear, sadness, anger, and shame. How intense is the feeling? For example, the spectrum of anger includes mild annoyance, exasperation, irritation, resentment, hostility, and rage. Can you notice more than one emotion present at a time, especially the softer, more vulnerable feelings beneath any angry ones? (See the box on self-observation.)

In order to name your deeper feelings, relax and let your awareness sink down into younger layers of your being; see what might be similar there to your current situation, perhaps intensifying your reactions to present-day events with your children or mate. For example, feeling let down by your partner could be amplified by experiences in which important people were not there for you as a child. Much as every child is innocent and good, you are innocent and good yourself at your roots. Try to bring an attitude of compassion for yourself to all that you feel. Sometimes there will be a memory or image of some episode, but often there will simply be a sense of a feeling that has a young quality to it.

Paradoxically, experiencing your feelings fully helps you let them go. Try to own them, even the most difficult ones, inside your mind: *This is my anger, my sadness, my frustration. I'm out of my mind with worry about the baby. I really do feel let down by my partner. I feel embarrassed trying to pump milk at work.* You let yourself feel bad for a moment in order to feel good for a long time. (For an extended experience of expressing emotions within your own mind, try the "safe room" exercise in Appendix B.)

Of course, it's hard to claim your feelings as your own if you can't accept them. As one mother put it: *The worst part of it is I get mad at myself for how I'm feeling. This is supposed to be a happy time, so I must be doing something wrong if I'm grouchy or sad.* Often our reactions to our experience are more stressful than the experience itself, like feeling ashamed of being needy, or getting mad at yourself for becoming irritated once again. We suffer *that* we suffer, wishing that our experiences were different or feeling guilty about them. For example, one mother said: *I feel mad at Tyler for making me mad. I just want to feel happy with him, not irritated. I feel upset about being upset so much!* Instead, see if you can bring compassion to your feelings. They occur for real reasons, triggered by hard situations today or by the painful residue of difficult experiences you had as an innocent child, and they are not your fault.

Imagine bringing the same compassion to yourself that you'd have for someone else who's upset, like your child or a dear friend. You can be a dear friend yourself to the distressed parts within you.

There is nothing shameful about a feeling itself, and accepting it is not the same as acting on it. When a person resists her feelings through suppression, denial, or minimization, they keep sticking around, like a preschooler pounding on a closed door. But when you accept them and express them to yourself, the door opens, the pounding stops, and the feelings can move on.

Self-Observation

At any moment, you can separate from the flow of your experiences and observe them like a neutral witness, as if a part of you has stepped out of the movie of your life and now sits ten rows back, watching the drama on the screen and describing it to yourself: *OK, there I'm getting really irritated with Jesse's whining, I'm thinking it's hopeless, I really wish he would hush up, a part of me would like to swat him, I feel bad about that, I'm getting into that whole thing about how I'm a crappy parent, it makes me really tense.* Rather than *being* an experience, *have* it. When you step back to observe it, you are still experiencing it but it's now less stressful.

Try to observe your experiences in little snapshots while you're on the go or by taking a few minutes to tune in to yourself. Notice the details in your inner world, especially the body sensations, emotions, and desires—not just the chatter of verbal thoughts. Notice the layering in your consciousness, with softer, younger, more fundamental material underneath more angry, adult, or superficial preoccupations.

Notice how your experiences are continually changing. Most of the flotsam and jetsam in your stream of consciousness is probably not that significant, but a largely automatic cascade of one thing triggering another. If anything disturbing comes along, you can watch it with interest and compassion, and then usually observe it becoming something else.

Expressing emotion symbolically. In this mode, you do express your feelings outwardly, yet still not directly to the person they concern. The most obvious way is to write them down without editing or censoring yourself, remembering that no one will see these words but you. If you like, you could write in large letters with crayons to bring out the younger feelings below the surface, or use your nondominant hand. In a more structured way, you could draft multiple letters to a person (*not* to send) in which you focus on different feelings such as hurt or anger. You could then release your writings through physical action, such as by throwing them away, cutting them into pieces and flushing them down a toilet, or burning them and scattering the ashes. As you do this, you may want to speak some words of release, in your mind or out loud, such as *I am letting go of these feelings. As this paper burns, my anger is turning into smoke. I am cleansed inside. Goodbye, feelings!*

Or you could draw pictures—which is about exploring and expressing your inner world, not worrying about whether you've made good art. Take a moment to get a sense of what you are feeling and then let it flow through you and onto the page. Don't be concerned if there seems to be no logic to it. Let your hand movements be big and free. If it helps, you can speak out loud or make sounds while drawing. You can be completely unstructured or abstract, or you can do loosely representational drawings focused on subjects such as you in relation to another person. You can also combine pictures and words, such as a cartoon of a typical argument with your spouse, with balloons over the heads that show what each person is thinking.

Venting out loud is another form of symbolic expression. Please do this only when you are alone and no one can hear you (especially your kids!). The shower may be a good place, the top of a hill, or inside your car (as long as you can continue to drive safely). If you feel you are losing control or getting lost in a negative emotion, stop venting and do what you need to do to calm down. You can also vent through physical action, not words. You could tear paper, smash your pillow against your bed over and over, hit something soft, or jump up and down. Again, do this while alone and where no one can see or hear you, and be sure not to hurt yourself.

Finally, you could express yourself to someone else. Pick a trustworthy person, tell them your purpose in talking, and ask for whatever would make you feel safe, such as a promise to keep things confidential. You are not looking for advice, but for someone to hear you out so you can move on, nor do you want to fan the flames of your feelings, since your purpose is release. As you speak, try to sense that the feelings are leaving you, that your listener is drawing them out of you and receiving them. You can ask the listener to help you let go by saying things like *I got it, I hear you, yes, OK.*

Riding the Wave of Desire

There is a collision, often many times a day, between a parent's desires and the needs and realities of life with children. In addition to being lovable, fascinating, delightful, etc., kids can be . . . frustrating. You desperately want them to eat their supper and all they want to do is smear it in their hair. You want them to come here but they crawl away, or to hug Grandpa but they hide behind your legs. Children grab hold of your life, and then just by being kids, they oblige you to do one thing after another that could be a million miles away from your personal preference at the moment.

Any desire is like a wave that starts small in the mind, builds to a crest of intensity, and then subsides when it is fulfilled or you decide to let it go. When your wants are frustrated, especially on a regular basis, this naturally creates stress. Relief comes from knowing how to ride the wave of wanting lightly, and how to let go when it's time to move on.

There is nothing wrong with wanting itself, whether it's your most fleeting wishes or deepest values. At bottom, every one of your wants is positive, even if some might be expressed in a problematic way. For example, Rick had a client who was troubled by a compulsive need to have her five-year-old in sight at all times. Of course, her compulsion was founded on a healthy desire to keep her child safe, and, over time, she learned more reasonable ways to feel secure about his safety. At its core, her want was always positive.

But trouble comes when we cling too tightly to our wants. Children bring one surprise after another, disrupting order, cleanliness, schedules, and plans. They also make you more dependent on others who have agendas of their own, such as your partner or childcare providers. As a mother, you probably have less control over your life than you've ever had, and accepting this fact can help you feel less stressed. As a mother of four-year-old twins told Rick: *I'm not obsessive, but I like things tidy and I like knowing what's going to happen. The clutter and constant changes drove me crazy for a long time. Finally I realized I had to give up. Now I insist on my bedroom being neat and just do what I can with the rest of the house. I try to remember that the big picture is going fine with the boys and not get too caught up in the little details. And I use work as a refuge: At least there, things happen on time!*

Pursuing healthy wants brings success and provides a positive model for children. On the other hand, some wants are unattainable or inappropriate, and we need to let them go and move on to a different plan. Here's how:

Step back. You can observe a want just like you can observe a thought or feeling. That bit of distance alone can lower the dial on your stress meter. You'll probably notice many desires, some nested within others, some pulling in opposite directions. Every aspect of this bubbling stew is normal, including the wilder wants all of us have. In particular, you'll see how wants that are rooted in early life experiences can be transferred into the present; for example, you may find yourself yearning for things from your partner that you missed getting from your father. This process of "transference" occurs for everyone, but it is intensified when you have kids because you are drawn into the kind of situations you experienced as a child. The problem is that wants that are normal for a child—like being the center of someone's universe—just aren't going to be fulfilled to the same degree in adult relationships. Through self-observation, you can separate the unattainable wants of your childhood from the adult wants that have a chance at being satisfied.

Relax. Usually, the more important the want, the more we feel it in the body. So when you relax, wanting can become less insistent.

Release feelings about not fulfilling the want. Notice any feelings of frustration or disappointment about not getting what you want. You can let go of these much like you would any other emotion, using the techniques described in the previous section. Try to be kind to yourself about your wants, especially if they come from your childhood. The stronger these young desires are, the more likely it is that they were not treated with attention and kindness when you were little. They really should have been; every child deserves that kind of care. If you take an attitude toward them that is dismissive, cold, or shaming, you are doing to yourself what should *not* have been done to you in the first place. Instead, try to be like a good mom to the young parts within you, sympathetic and understanding.

Release the want itself. You could remind yourself of the reasons why it is not realistic or wise to attain it, perhaps even writing a note to yourself. You can say goodbye to it in your mind, out loud, in a letter to yourself, or to another person. You could imagine that it is draining out of you like water into sand. As a last resort, sometimes we just have to accept that a particular want will never be fulfilled, and it brings peace to find a kind of surrender, a giving up and complete letting go.

Move on to a new plan. This might be a small matter—like taking a break from trying to shovel peas into your toddler—or a fundamental shift in your deepest values. You can help the new plan feel concrete by saying it to yourself, writing it down, or telling someone else. You could also help yourself feel good about it by focusing on its benefits or imagining it going well.

Insights That Free You

Untrue, illogical, or overly negative thoughts increase your stress—and insight into them is like waking up from a bad dream, usually to good news, as one mother found out: *I got a message at work that the day care staff had phoned me. I called them and called them, but their line was always busy, so I left and drove over. It's true, I usually assume the worst. I was sure Jasmine had gotten hurt, and I worried about all the horrible possibilities the whole way. When I got there, they said she was fine, they'd had some trouble with their phones, and they just wanted to tell me they'd gotten our payment last week. What a relief!*

Reframing stresses as opportunities. Let's say your 15-month-old kicks and thrashes when you try to put him in his car seat. It's natural to feel frustrated and angry. But it's also possible to regard the situation as an opportunity for learning new skills, developing greater patience, enjoying a feeling of accomplishment, deepening your sense of compassion and love, and even experiencing spiritual growth. Seeing both sides of the coin—the challenges *and* the opportunities—will improve both your well-being and how you cope.

Talking back to the voice in your head. Just because a thought arises in your mind does not mean it's worth believing. You can catch the unrealistic beliefs that are making you stressed and replace them with true, logical, and positive ones. Many studies have found that this positive self-talk is one of the most powerful ways to cope with stress. In essence, you are sticking up for yourself inside your own mind by focusing on the objective facts, defending yourself against unfair attacks, and giving encouragement. (See the box for some of the beliefs that can help a mother cope well with stress.)

Beliefs That Help Mothers Cope

The real problem here is just ______. It is a hassle, but not life or death.

Things could have gone much worse.

It's not permanent.

Things will get better.

I have handled this in the past and I can handle it again.

I will figure something out.

I have resources all around me.

I can create more resources if I need to.

Determination will get me through this problem, just like it always has.

Even if I can't change the situation, I'll grow from it.

I am a good person.

I am doing my best.

Most of the time, you'll stand up to stressful thoughts inwardly, within your own head. But it can also help to put it in writing: Just draw a line down the center of a piece of paper; write an untrue, illogical, or negative thought on the left side; and then list two or more true, logical, and positive ones on the right side. Whether it's in your mind or on paper, try to make a strong case for yourself, arguing actively with negative beliefs and refusing to let them defeat you. With practice, you'll be talking back to them quickly and naturally.

Let's try this method with some different categories of stressful thinking. When you start becoming able to recognize the *type* of thought that's raising your blood pressure, you've got a jump start on letting go of it.

- *Exaggerating the problem*

NEGATIVE THOUGHT	POSITIVE ALTERNATIVES
Babysitters never work out.	So far, there's been only one problem. Even if a babysitter doesn't show up, all it means is that Bob and I don't get to go out to dinner. Maybe an older person would be more responsible than a teenage babysitter.

- *Focusing on the negative*

NEGATIVE THOUGHT	POSITIVE ALTERNATIVES
The preschool teacher said Johnny was "rambunctious."	She also said he was sweet, smart, helpful, friendly, creative, and liked by everyone. Almost everything she said was positive.

Even if he is "rambunctious," nobody has complained about Johnny being aggressive, wild, or mean.

Outside of preschool, he is well behaved.

So what if he gets rambunctious? That's normal for a three-year-old!

- *Discounting the positive*

NEGATIVE THOUGHT	POSITIVE ALTERNATIVES
People at work look down on me since I took time off for the baby.	Most of my coworkers are friendly; they like me. If people like me, it means I am likable. No one is forcing them to like me. Every woman at work who's a mom has let me know she thought it was great I took the time off.

- *Dooming the future*

NEGATIVE THOUGHT	POSITIVE ALTERNATIVES
I'm going to have to put the baby in day care 40 hours a week because I'm never going to find a good part-time job.	Good part-time jobs do exist. I've seen them advertised. I know people who have them, and they are less on the ball than I am.

I've only been looking for three weeks.

I can try changing my résumé, working with a personnel agency, or doing temporary work.

Whenever I have stayed determined in the past, I have always succeeded.

✦ *Overgeneralizing*

NEGATIVE THOUGHT	POSITIVE ALTERNATIVES
Men don't listen.	I can remember times when men listened to me. OK, my dad didn't listen, but I chose my husband in part because he is different from my dad. My husband listened to me when ______ and when ______. I can talk to my husband about really hearing me out, and I couldn't do that with my dad.

- *Attributing negative intentions to others*

NEGATIVE THOUGHT	POSITIVE ALTERNATIVES
My kids are trying to manipulate me.	They are not old enough to be crafty and manipulative. They just want what they want and are trying to get it. It's OK that they are trying to persuade me, and it's OK for me to say no.

Being mindful of stressful thoughts. Through paying attention to your thoughts in daily life, you'll get better at recognizing the ones that cause you extra stress—and then letting them go. We also recommend you try meditation: In addition to being wonderfully relaxing and a proven method of lowering blood pressure, it's a great way to practice observing the stream of thoughts and feelings, like an endless train passing by, without jumping on board (see the box).

Meditation

Meditation has been practiced in various forms for thousands of years, and you may already have some experience with it. If not, we can suggest a simple yet fundamental method:

Find a comfortable place to sit in an upright position, perhaps on a pillow or a chair. Set aside 15 minutes or more if you can; even five minutes can be helpful, though you will generally go deeper the longer you sit. Try meditating for one minute if much longer seems overwhelming.

With your eyes open or closed, take a big breath. Roll your head around, or otherwise adjust your position to feel comfortable. Sweep your attention through your body and relax any tension.

Breathing in and out through your nose, focus on the physical sensations of the breath, your belly rising and falling, the air going in and out of your throat, the coolness of the exhalation on your upper lip. Let your focus on your breath be a kind of anchor that enables you to witness the waves of passing thoughts and feelings without getting caught up in them. You need not struggle with this stream or try to control it. You are only being with it, letting it come and go, focusing on your breath.

If your mind wanders, that's normal; simply return your attention to the breath. It may help center you to count your breaths for a while, from one to ten and then start over; if you lose track before you get to ten, just start the count again.

As the minutes pass, you may find your thoughts quieting and a sense of spacious peacefulness emerging, like the way sediment in a pond settles to reveal clear water. But if this doesn't happen at first, it's alright: It will with practice and time.

When it's time to end your meditation, you can return gently to the outer world, sitting for a moment longer with your eyes open, breathing, letting the experience linger. As you meditate more regularly, this sense of peace will stay with you throughout your day.

Pinning down the sources of stressful thoughts. You've probably noticed that stressful thoughts bubble up from particular sources in your mind, such as the inner critic that often gets louder when a woman has children. Many of these sources lurk in the shadows, outside your conscious awareness. Shining a light on where a thought comes from helps you judge its credibility, much like you'd be skeptical of a news bulletin about the wonderful health benefits of a particular brand of infant formula when you find out it comes from the manufacturer; thoughts from certain sources in your mind should be considered guilty until proven innocent! As soon as you identify where a stressful thought comes from, you have a head start on letting it go. Sources of stressful thoughts include:

- **Beliefs about motherhood.** You could look back on the hopes and dreams for motherhood and family you had during the pregnancy of your first child. Were any of those unrealistic and worth letting go of today? You might also list, in your mind or on paper, some of the beliefs about how a mother *should* be that give you stress, such as *A good mother never gets angry at her children* or *I should always look as put together as my mother did.*
- **Temperament and mood.** If you tend to be cautious or anxious, your thoughts might overstate problems and underemphasize how well you can cope. If you are inclined to depression or sadness, your thoughts are more likely to contain themes of loss, defeat, and helplessness. If you often feel aggressive or irritable, you'll have more thoughts about how other people are challenging or threatening. When you understand these things about yourself, you can routinely put in a correction factor, like *I know I'm in a bad mood today, so of course everything looks like a huge problem. But it's really not.*
- **Subpersonalities.** The mind is like a big committee—though sometimes it may seem more like a zoo! All of these "subpersonalities" are trying to help you, but some of them just increase

your stress, like the one that says your home has to look perfect before anyone can come over. By understanding your subpersonalities, you'll be more able to detach from those that wear you down. You can tune in to a subpersonality by imagining that part of yourself and then ask what it thinks, feels, or wants—as if it were a person in its own right. If you talk with it respectfully, its views and agenda will usually become less demanding, but if you argue with it, it will dig in further or go underground. You can also imagine or write out a dialogue between two subpersonalities—such as the part of you that is ambitious for a career and the part of you that wants to stay home with your child—or even among several parts of yourself, such the critic, vulnerable child, and nurturing parent, as you can see in the dialogue in the box.

Sample Dialogue with the Inner Critic, Vulnerable Child, and Nurturing Parent

Critic: *Listen to that baby cry! You messed up again. As usual!*

Vulnerable Child: *I'm sorry, sorry, sorry.*

Critic: *Quit whining. You're pathetic.*

Nurturing Parent: *Hold on here. She didn't make Susie cry. It's not her fault. Susie is just fussing like a normal baby.*

Vulnerable Child: *Yeah!*

Critic: *Yes, she did. She never feeds her right.*

Nurturing Parent: *No way. The doctor said she was doing a great job.*

Critic: *It doesn't matter. It's her job to do everything right.*

Nurturing Parent: *EVERYTHING?! That's nuts. She's doing great as a new mom.*

Critic: *I'm just trying to get her to be perfect.*

Nurturing Parent: *She is a perfectly good mother already. Every mother has to learn things, and it's only harder when she is getting yelled at by you.*

Critic: *She still shouldn't have let the baby cry.*

Nurturing Parent: *She absolutely did not "let" the baby cry! All babies cry, no matter how "perfect" their mothers are. Susie just woke up and wants some love. See, she's settling down; Carol is really helping her. She's doing a great job. As usual! I know you're trying to help, but you're too extreme about it!*

- **Beliefs from childhood.** We all formed many ideas and expectations when we were little that we still tend to apply unconsciously to ourselves and the world. For example, one of Jan's clients was the oldest of 11 children, and it has been hard for her *not* to assume that everything in her family today was her responsibility. It can feel wonderfully freeing to realize how a belief from your childhood just doesn't apply today: The thinking of a child draws conclusions from only a handful of individuals; it sees oneself as small and weak compared to others; it overemphasizes negative experiences (a single scary experience with a dog is more memorable than 99 pleasant ones); and it makes all-or-nothing rules that oversimplify the complexity of adult life. Today, you can truly afford to let go of those beliefs. You have so much more choice about who you are with, and you have so many more ways to take care of yourself. As a result, the world is safer, people are kinder and more trustworthy, and you are more capable than you've probably thought.

Taking in the Good

> *I see women's spirits getting weaker and weaker when they don't fill their pitchers up, when they don't recharge.*
>
> Shoshana Bennett, PhD, Founder,
> Postpartum Assistance for Mothers

Now that you've learned how to let go of stressful experiences, we can explore how to replace them with positive ones. Every day has dozens of little opportunities—such as moments of pleasure, achievement, or love—to replenish yourself psychologically. Each of these is an oasis where you can rest briefly and refuel yourself for the challenges ahead.

Letting yourself enjoy the good moments does not take anything away from anyone else. Try to notice if you have any reluctance to linger with a nice experience, such as thinking you are supposed to be on the go every second. Or resistance to accepting a compliment, as if that would be vain, or *If they really knew the truth about me they wouldn't be so nice.* Or discomfort with receiving recognition or love, as if that would make you seem needy. You can use the methods you've already learned to let go of these reactions as you would any other negative thought or feeling.

Throughout your day, really try to pay attention to positive events. For example, notice everything you're accomplishing. Or has your child been especially cute, your partner acted supportively, or someone praised your work? Try to infuse ordinary events with positive meaning. For instance, it is possible to see making a meal or folding laundry as gifts of love that can make you feel good about yourself, not merely repetitive chores.

We're not talking about million-dollar moments, but the small change of everyday life. In a fundamental sense, the person you are is the distillation of all the experiences you've ever had. By consciously putting new, good ones in the emotional memory bank each day, you build up an increasingly positive balance.

So when a tasty dish is set before you, dive in with a big spoon! As your day unfolds, make sure that positive events register as positive *experiences*. Stay with those experiences a few seconds or minutes longer than you normally would. Let your body relax around the good feelings, be filled with them, and soak them up like a sponge. If you like, you could imagine that they are being placed in a treasure chest in your heart, and you can take them out and feel them again any time you want.

You could also set aside specific times for reflecting on the good things in your life. For example, you might like to do a brief meditation at the end of each day in which you look back for happy moments and successes, and then allow these to sink in. Or you could do this through writing in a journal (see the box).

A Journal for a Mother

Many mothers have found that keeping a journal is a wonderful way to have a record of this unique time in their lives. It's also a good way to carve out a specific time for yourself each day. It might even help you work through a problem or issue. You may already be experienced with keeping a journal. If not, here are some suggestions:

- You can write in a physical journal or on a computer. Make sure your privacy will be respected so you can express yourself freely. And try not to be judgmental about what you say or how it all comes out.

- In addition to writing about whatever comes to mind, you might like to regularly reflect on questions such as *What did I accomplish today? What was enjoyable? What's one way I was a loving, skillful mother? What did I learn or how did I grow?*
- Explore different styles of self-expression, such as poetry, drawing, dialogues between parts of yourself or between you and another person, letters that you will never send to your partner, mother, or others, and so on.
- Some people like to reread what they wrote that day, or periodically look back at entries from months or years before.
- There are many lovely books about journaling, such as *Keeping a Journal You Love* by Sheila Bender, *Leaving a Trace* by Alexandra Johnson, and *The Artist's Way* by Julia Cameron.

Out with the Old, In with the New

Going a step further, you could actively dislodge old, bad experiences from their places in emotional memory by replacing them with new, good experiences. One mother offered this example: *Growing up, people told me I wouldn't amount to much. So when Jorge's preschool teacher told me I was a good mom, I just brushed it off. "No," she said, "I really mean it. I've watched you with him for a year and I can see that you are really good with him." We were alone in her office, she put her hand on my arm, and I started to cry. I was embarrassed, but she was so sincere I decided to believe her. Something melted inside me, and I realized that I've done at least one good thing in my life, and I have felt better about myself ever since.*

All you have to do is be aware of both experiences at the same time—the present, positive one and the old, unpleasant one—and let the new one be a more powerful experience than the old. Then you'll have an internal sense of the good, current experience dissolving and replacing the painful, old one, of finally getting fed where you are hungry inside. You might be giving yourself today some of what you didn't get—but should have gotten—as a child.

In particular, try experiments in which you do something that challenges a negative belief, and observe the results. For example, if you normally feel nervous about being assertive because deep down you expect to be punished for it in some way, you could try being one notch more direct, blunt, or forceful with your partner, a friend, or a coworker. If the experiment goes badly (but make sure it's a fair one!), maybe the old belief is true after all. If it goes well—which is what usually happens—then let the good news sink in. This process is probably the single most effective method of personal growth we know, and every day brings new opportunities to use it.

Creating Positive Experiences

In addition to taking in the good experiences that naturally come your way, you can create new ones.

A regular personal practice. Options include spiritual or inspirational reading, meditation, yoga, prayer, writing a poem, attending twelve-step meetings, knitting, art, crafts, exercise, a peaceful walk with the dog, or simply a long bath. Whatever form it takes, a personal practice creates new experiences—sometimes profound ones—that are innately nourishing. Perhaps you had a practice that fell by the wayside once children arrived; if so, it could be time to take it up again or find something else that's doable in the life you have today. And if you've never had one, we strongly suggest you find something that you can regularly do for yourself.

Rather than taking on something too ambitious that fades out in a few weeks, it's better to have a modest practice that you can stick with most days. Some mothers wake up a little early in order to have a quiet time to themselves in the morning, and that might mean making sure you get to bed at a sensible hour the night before. Your partner may be willing to take care of the kids at a regular time while you do your practice; you could exchange the favor, or he might simply be happy to support you in this way with nothing needed in return.

Especially after kids come along, you have to make your practice matter, or it will be pushed aside. Finding other people with a similar interest—such as in a church, reading group, or art class—is one way to help yourself stay committed, plus it enriches the whole experience.

Reaching out to others. Studies have shown that one of the most powerful ways to reduce stress—especially for a woman—is to have the experience of feeling connected to another person. Try to create friendships with other people—especially other mothers—who you'd feel comfortable talking with when your stress meter starts redlining. Perhaps you could think of someone who's called you during a hair-on-fire moment; she would probably be kind and supportive if you texted her when you're feeling frazzled. You don't have to talk about whatever it is that's stressing you—just being able to chat might help you feel a whole lot better in a few minutes.

Since raising a child today is often quite isolating, especially if you're a stay-at-home mom, it helps to think systematically about how you could connect with other people. An obvious place to start is with your relatives; for example, having a baby brings many women closer to their own mothers. On the other hand, relatives can also meddle and criticize. Paradoxically, knowing that you can close the door to unwanted comments or advice enables you to open up to relationships with your family and in-laws. If someone starts saying something you'd rather not hear, remember that it's *your* child, that you understand him or her better than anyone else in the world, and that your parenting values may differ from those of the other person. You can listen politely if you want, or if necessary say something like, "That's interesting, but I've decided to raise my child a little differently."

Neighbors are another good source of companionship and practical support. If you're not meeting people in the ordinary flow of your day, you might need to go out of your way to strike up a conversation. You could invite neighbors over for a casual meal, or see if there's one of those neighborhood associations that are common in many areas.

Playgroups, babysitting co-ops, and mothers' clubs are great ways to meet other parents. To connect with one of these, ask around, look online—or start one yourself! Preschool parent associations, sports activities (such as soccer, T-ball, gymnastics, martial arts), or youth programs are similar opportunities to get to know new people.

Of course, you can meet people in situations that don't have anything to do with parenting. These include religious and civic organizations, charities, environmental groups, and so on. Fundamentally, whether you're shy or outgoing, there are many ways develop a greater sense of community with others.

Scheduling good times. If you do not make time for the things you especially enjoy, they will get crowded out by the world and other people. Even small moments for yourself can make a big difference. For instance, a patient of Jan's told her: *After I've dropped Jason off at preschool, I'll come home, make some eggs and toast for myself, and then sit down and eat my breakfast alone. It's just this little ritual I perform for myself. It seems so basic, but what makes it special is doing it in peace and taking the time to really enjoy it, instead of gulping down breakfast cereal with the kids at the table.*

You could make a deal with your partner about breaks for each other, perhaps for half an hour to yourself in the evening, or for several hours each weekend. For example, one of Ricki's patients has a monthly dinner with three other women.

Or you could make sure that there are times with your kids that are especially enjoyable for *you*. Make a mental list of what you most like doing with your children, and go out of your way to do those activities on a regular basis. Plus dream up a wish list of things you'd *like* to do with your kids, and then do at least some of them. It doesn't have to be a big-ticket item. At a talk Rick gave, one mother laughed when she said, *My dream is to go shopping with my kids . . . while my husband comes along to watch them!*

> *There is no pleasure in having nothing to do; the fun is in having lots to do and not doing it.*
>
> Mary Little

Focusing on being, rather than doing. Sure, there's a lot to do, but you might be running around like the Energizer Bunny much more than you need to. Maybe you've got a perfectionistic streak, or you think you need to "make it up to my child" if you feel guilty about needing to work, or you might stay busy as a way to avoid certain feelings. Maybe you find yourself constantly checking your phone or social media accounts, which keeps you half-listening, half-present.

Happily, though, every so often, you get a chance to stop all that doing for a bit. Perhaps the inbox is empty, the baby's asleep, the bills are paid. The urgency of the daily round falls away, and a quiet fills the air. Your thoughts slow down, no longer grabbed and jostled by tasks. You are present in *this* moment, not worried about the future. You feel freer, less bound by your burdens, less limited by your roles. The edges soften. Each breath comes like a wave on the seashore, rising and falling, the ocean abiding. There is peace, contentment, warmth, and happiness, just here, just as you are. In this state of mind, you can do tasks as well, but the pot gets stirred or the phone answered in a way that feels much less stressful.

As you relax, you will usually experience a growing sense of your innermost being. This core of the self is a fundamental property of the human nervous system. It may be overlooked, but it cannot be tainted or destroyed. All you can do is uncover it and allow it to come forward into your daily life. It is always loving, peaceful, and wise, a bottomless well of clarity and strength, detached from the daily craziness, a refuge of nourishment and quiet humor, your own true self.

Essential being is an extraordinary resource for anyone, but especially for a mother. In the turbulence of the typical day, your innermost being is a place to watch the storms within you (or between you and others) swell and crash and blow over. As you rest in being, compassion comes naturally for family and friends and others—and for yourself. Compassion lets you hold your own sorrows and pain with a tender concern, helping you remember that you are doing the best you can, that you have already come through a lot simply to stand here today.

For many people, their essential nature is also a window within to the Divine, and they feel most available to God or some other higher power when grounded in their deepest being. One does not need to believe this in order to reap the benefits of cultivating a sense of one's being. But you may feel that the spark of the Divine is what gives your essence its light, providing the most profound form of nurturance in your life.

Whatever your spiritual orientation may be, including none at all, a child can help awaken a sense of your innermost being. Children arrive, in the words of William Wordsworth, "trailing clouds of glory." The eyes of a child are radiant with a mysterious illumination, and a mother can always replenish herself by letting in that light.

The Enjoyment of Being

You might like to consider these questions:

When you are busy doing one thing after another, what do you feel like? Energized, numb, tense, driven, productive, weary?

What inside you draws you into the role of a doer? A sense of duty? Habit? A reluctance to ask others to do more? Concern about what people might think if you do less?

How does "doing" feel different from "being"?

You also might like to try some of these suggestions:

Consider your worth to others in terms of who you are *rather than what you do.*

Try being more of a benign and loving presence who steps back and does less while others do more of the problem-solving and task accomplishment.

Try an experiment for a week: Set aside a time each day, ideally 20 minutes or more, when you can just be with your child without trying to get anything done. What happens, and how does it feel?

Ask each person in your family to start doing one small thing that you've done in the past, so that you can do one thing less.

> I don't think the quiet mind is very far away for anybody.

> I don't think the place of stillness is very far away for anybody.
> It doesn't matter whether you're chopping wood or sitting on a meditation cushion.
> It doesn't matter whether you're in intensive retreat or you're living a very creative and vital life.
> What's important is that your home is in stillness.
>
> Christina Feldman

Key Ideas from This Chapter

- Your inner experience matters in its own right, plus nurturing yourself is the foundation of caring for your children.
- You can be active in your own mind, ultimately in charge of it, like the skillful rider of a horse.
- The little moments of stress really add up over time, so do small things throughout the day to keep your stress meter out of the red zone.
- Routinely focus on letting go of stress in your body, mental images, emotions, desires, and thoughts.
- Try to accept your inner experience for what it is. Accepting it is not the same as acting on it.
- Reflect on how your childhood is affecting you today; bring compassion to the young parts of yourself; try to sort apart the intensified "young" reactions from the more moderate, here-and-now ones; try to let go of the deepest level of any distressing feelings, like making sure you get the tip of the dandelion's root to prevent it from growing back.

- Try to let go of unrealistic expectations about the sort of mother you are "supposed" to be.
- Let positive experiences sink deeply into your emotional memory banks, soothing and even dislodging negative ones.
- Commit to one or more realistically doable daily practices, such as meditation or journaling, that nurture you and deepen your capacity to stand apart from the inevitable, endless ups and downs of your inner and outer worlds.
- If it's meaningful for you to do so, you can nourish and draw on a spiritual awareness in the middle of raising your family.

CHAPTER THREE

Transforming Painful Emotions

Insanity is hereditary—you get it from your children.
Sam Levinson

Chances are, parenthood has brought on some of the most intense feelings you've ever had. It's easy to feel that your emotions are happening *to* you, that you've got no control over them. But in fact, more than a century of psychological research has discovered numerous ways that you can consciously change the way you feel.

In this chapter, we'll be looking at ways to turn around feelings of sadness, anxiety, shame, and anger. Since motherhood can be both numbing and emotionally chaotic, it's sometimes hard to know *what* in the world you're actually feeling; take a look at the box for ways to identify your emotions. You can focus on the sections in this chapter that specifically relate to your emotional concerns, and within each one, we'll cover a range of difficulties, from mild to severe.

Identifying Your Emotions

Most of us experience just about every possible human emotion at least once a year, but some feelings are more of a "home base" to which we keep returning. The major emotions come in many shadings and intensities, and here is a kind of map of the emotional landscape:

- **Sadness:** Wistfulness, loss, regret, hurt, the blues, moping, sorrow, grief, melancholy, depression
- **Anxiety:** Worry, obsessing, compulsions, apprehension, fear, dread, panic, terror
- **Shame:** Self-consciousness, embarrassment, guilt, inadequacy, humiliation, worthlessness
- **Anger:** Frustration, irritation, annoyance, disdain or contempt, resentment, getting mad, rage, hatred

TURNING SADNESS INTO CONTENTMENT

Feelings of sadness, including depressed mood, are common among mothers. For example, approximately 10–12 percent will go through a clinical depression, and some studies have found that roughly half of the mothers of young children will suffer many of the symptoms of "persistent depressive disorder" (milder, but more chronic, depressive feelings). Everybody feels sad sometimes, just like some days are cloudy, and often your mood will change on its own. But when an emotional "low front" settles in and stays with you longer than it should, it's time to take a more active approach for the sake of your well-being.

Mourning Your Losses

Most mothers would say they're so very glad to have had their children. But that doesn't mean there aren't always losses as well, whether it's needing to put a hold on your career, less closeness with your partner, or simply never having a free hour to yourself. Many mothers find it hard to accept the feelings they have about such losses, sometimes because they fear being thought of as selfish or self-pitying. But if these understandable emotions are pushed down or minimized, then they will gradually drag your mood downward. We need to acknowledge our losses and allow the feelings that come with them to flow through the mind in a healthy way.

In the box, you'll find a six-step process for letting go of feelings of loss. You can do these steps in one sitting, or spread them out over several days or weeks. Feel free to adapt them to suit your own needs.

Mourning Past Losses

1. Look back at everything that has happened to you since conceiving your first child, including the changes in your body, career, friendships, finances, or marriage. Some of these changes have probably been gains, while others have been losses. Name your losses by listing them on paper or in your mind.
2. Write or think about the resources you've drawn on to cope with your losses. These include both external (e.g., friends, your mother, a savings account) as well as internal ones (e.g., patience, religious faith, self-knowledge).
3. Write or think about what you've learned or how you've grown from your losses.

4. Tell your partner or a trusted friend about your losses, how you coped, and how you've grown.
5. Imagine going into the safe room in your mind (see Appendix B) and really grieving your losses. Or if you like, find a comfortable place in your home or outdoors and grieve your losses out loud. Either way, try to really let yourself go, and sense that the whole experience of loss, and its related feelings, is flowing out of your body.
6. Imagine that the learning and growth related to your losses is sinking deeply into you, becoming a positive part of yourself.

Unlearning Helplessness

Because there's so much about mothering that's beyond anyone's control, a mom can begin to acquire a sense of "learned helplessness," a feeling of powerlessness and pessimism that lowers a person's energy and mood and makes her feel less confident about taking action to solve her problems. Studies have found that learned helplessness can be a major factor of depressed mood. The antidote is "learned optimism," an attitude that focuses on what you *can* do, on your successes, and on the future. With learned optimism, you develop realistically positive beliefs about yourself and your ability to make good things happen both out in the world and inside your own head. It's a self-fulfilling prophecy: When you think there's a good chance you'll succeed, you'll be more willing to make the efforts that will bring you success.

Therefore, try to pay attention every day to the good news about:

- **Yourself:** Your positive qualities and virtues, your honest efforts, the results you did indeed produce, and the ways you've been true to your deepest values, whatever the outcome. For example, if you're feeling blue about a hassle that won't go away with your in-laws about holidays with the children, you might focus on the patience you've shown, your sincere attempts to resolve the issue, the fact that at least everyone agreed to spend Christmas morning at your own home, and that you've always been motivated by wanting the best for your children.

- **The world:** The many good things that exist in your partner, extended family, friends and neighbors, other mothers, church or other institutions, libraries, online, and the natural world. For instance, if you feel stuck with a childcare situation that isn't working well, you could think about the many other forms and settings of childcare, including home day care, preschools, after-school programs, babysitting co-ops, swapping with other families, adjusting work schedules with your partner so there is more time to take care of your kids yourselves, or doing home day care yourself.
- **The future:** The positive scenarios that *could* realistically happen. Let's say that your three-year-old son is extremely stubborn and hates transitions. You could reflect on these facts: He will naturally become more flexible and easygoing over time, he will gravitate to friendships and situations that feel predictable and safe to him, and his strengths of determination and caution will bring him success in school and adult life.

Learned optimism is an attitude that focuses realistically on what is in your power to accomplish rather than what is not. As you recognize what you can actually succeed at, take some sort of *action*, either inside your mind or out in the world. When you're active, rather than passive, you'll both feel better and increase your capabilities. For example, if you have to get up at night with your colicky daughter, you can use the time to think through a problem at work or to come up with new funny songs to sing to her. If you're tired of changing diapers, but that situation is not changing any time soon, you could create a kind of game in your mind to see if you can stay relaxed in your body during a diaper change.

Talking Back to Sadness

Much research has shown that talking back to negative thoughts can lift a person's mood both in the moment and over time. You can identify thoughts and beliefs that bring you down and then come up with realistic and positive alternatives. Here are examples of several types of problematic thoughts to get you started.

- *Assuming there's nothing you can do*

NEGATIVE THOUGHT	POSITIVE ALTERNATIVES
I'm stuck in the house all day.	If the weather is OK, I can put Olivia in the stroller and go for a walk. If the weather is bad, we can go for a drive. Or go to a mall and window-shop. I could invite some other moms to come over. Even if I'm alone in the house with Olivia, I can make that better by playing music, watching a show, or calling a friend.

- *Feeling bad about things beyond your control*

NEGATIVE THOUGHT	POSITIVE ALTERNATIVES
Elijah keeps getting ear infections. I must be doing something wrong.	He's sick because of germs, not me. I've done everything the doctor has advised. I've taken really good care of him. I'm really sorry he's in pain. Feeling concerned and sympathetic is natural. But getting overwhelmed is not going to help him.

- *Assuming the future will be the same as the past*

NEGATIVE THOUGHT	POSITIVE ALTERNATIVES
My ex-husband left me, and I'm never going to find another partner again.	He's not the only man who has ever liked me; other men will like me too. I can put myself in situations where I'll meet good people. I don't have to sit home waiting for the phone to ring. My next relationship will be better than the last one since I will look for a different kind of man, and I will use what I learned from my marriage.

- *Brooding about a loss*

NEGATIVE THOUGHT	POSITIVE ALTERNATIVES
I'm missing important time with my son while I'm at work.	Being at work makes the time with him feel more precious.
	I know stay-at-home moms who sometimes get cranky with their kids because of all the time spent alone together.
	Perhaps I can figure out how to cut back my hours.

Finding Sources of Well-Being

Sad feelings are completely normal. And alongside them, you can also find genuine sources of gratitude, enjoyment, and contentment. Here are a few suggestions.

Enjoy your children. It's easy to get so caught up in the tasks of daily life that you miss opportunities to enjoy your children. But there are always moments each day when you could take the time for an extra cuddle or linger a few seconds longer when they're being extra cute. You can also plan activities that you particularly enjoy yourself, something besides knocking down a tower of blocks over and over.

Accept the changes in your life. There's a kind of wishful thinking in our society that says a woman can simply graft motherhood onto her old life. But if you don't accommodate to the changes that come with children, it's like trying to hold back the tide. For example, you might find that you can't raise young children with the same attitude that propelled you forward in your career. It's just not possible. Raising children takes up *space* in a person's life. It has to replace some things and push others to the edges, especially during the years when children are little.

You can help yourself by seeing what, if any, wishful thoughts still linger in your mind about somehow returning to business as usual. Or unrealistic expectations about motherhood that you are straining to live up to. Or any ongoing underestimates of the new needs or priorities that have come with children. If you find any of these, you can use the methods you learned in the previous chapter, such as talking back to unrealistic expectations or letting in the reality of new needs.

Laugh away the tears. Sometimes it's so awful it's funny. One parent told Rick: *I'd had a string of bad days, and this was another one. Just as I got the baby to sleep, I heard a noise in the kitchen. My boyfriend was on the phone in our bedroom, so no one was watching Tucker. I found him squirting ketchup on the floor and finger painting with it. He looked up and smiled proudly! It was so ridiculous, I started laughing and laughing. We had to clean it up, but it was the first time I'd felt good in a week.*

You can draw on your sense of humor in numerous ways. Just taking a few big breaths while you smile gently can improve your attitude. You could try to spend more time with lighthearted friends or coworkers, scroll through your favorite funny Instagram accounts, or read a humorous book about motherhood. Perhaps imagine the weirder moments in your day as if they were scenes in a sitcom with a laugh track. None of these is a miracle cure, but over time they can help. And it's good for your kids to hear you laugh!

"Top Ten Topics for Future Presentations at Our Mothers' Club"

This was a tongue-in-cheek list of future topics offered to the membership of a mother's club:

10. Breasts—Here Today, Gone Tomorrow

9. Hips—Gone Today, Here Tomorrow

8. Time-Saver—How to Starch Business Suits So You Can Sleep in Them
7. Dinner in a Diaper—New Product Idea
6. 365 Meals You Can Make with One Hand
5. Sex After Kids—When, Where, How, and *Why?*
4. How to Turn Spit-Up Stains into Fashion Statements
3. Styling Techniques for Unwashed Hair
2. Baby Talk—I Understand It, and It Scares Me
1. How to Stop the Crying—Yours!

Shine a light. Bright light, particularly sunshine, can lift your mood, especially if you get gloomy during dark winters. Try to spend more time outside during daylight, clean dingy windows, or pull the drapes back. Even brighter lights might help.

Get exercise. Regular aerobic exercise (ideally three or more times a week, half an hour each time) will increase the serotonin in your brain and lift your mood.

Keep good company. Few things can lift your mood like the empathy, kindness, and emotional support of others; for suggestions on how to connect with others while raising a family, see page 75. If you are wrestling with a loss, look into a support group; for example, most counties have groups for women who have become single mothers or who have lost a child. (Support from your partner is covered in chapters 6, 7, and 8.) Online communities can help you feel less alone, but curate them carefully. If a feed leaves you feeling judged, less than others, or anxious, it's not support—it's added stress. And above all, really try to notice the support that's actually there for you, including all the little things; studies have found that *perceiving* support is a key to alleviating mental and physical distress.

Have some fun. A mother tells this story: *My sister came to town and watched the kids, and Joaquin and I went out to dinner. Afterwards, on a whim, we stepped into a local jazz club. We had a great time, and it reminded me that a whole world exists outside of shopping for diapers or commuting to work.*

How much fun did you have this week? If it wasn't much, make a list of activities you enjoyed before you had children, and think about how you could start doing some of them again. It's usually surprisingly easy; you just have to make a commitment to yourself: *I've always loved riding fast downhill on my bike . . . the feeling of the wind and the freedom is so exhilarating! But when I got pregnant, the bike went into the garage. Every so often, after Carson was born, I'd think wistfully about going for a ride, but there never seemed to be enough time. One weekend, though, I was feeling just blah, and sick and tired of being blah. I just decided to get the bike out and to heck with everything else. Well, when I got going again, that old thrill came right back. I couldn't stop smiling. My whole mood changed. Since then, I try to ride every day, even if it's only down the street and back. It's so little, but it makes me feel so much better.*

Make a contribution. If your mood is slumping, putting out even more energy is challenging. Nonetheless, by finding some form of community service—such as volunteering once a month to serve meals at a shelter or tutoring a young child—you'll feel good about yourself, spend time with other people, be distracted from your own difficulties, and even access a kind of self-nurturing source inside as you nurture others.

See the good that is also true. When you appreciate what you have, rather than longing for or grumbling about what you don't, feelings of contentment nurture you from the inside out. A mother told Rick a story about straightening up her six-year-old's bedroom one day. The usual debris was everywhere and she was grumbling to herself about him, why didn't he pick up after all her reminders, she was sick of housework, he would probably just clutter it all up again, and so on. Then she happened to turn over a *National Geographic* magazine whose cover showed people walking through the wreckage of a town after a hurricane. In an instant her perspective changed as she compared her own life to that of the people in the photograph. She suddenly appreciated the dirty socks on the floor because they meant her children had clothes to wear at all. She thought about the other good things her family had, how they were safe and could enjoy life. Days later, when she was feeling down, she thought back on that evening and was grateful for her good fortune, which immediately helped her feel better.

> *Parents are often so busy with the physical rearing of children that they miss the glory of parenthood, just as the grandeur of trees is lost when raking leaves.*
>
> Marceline Cox

Sprinkling moments of thankfulness throughout your day is like taking sips of cool water while working under a hot sun. In daily life, you could try to notice the little occasions of beauty, pleasure, or growth. You could say some kind of grateful blessing at a meal. You could tell another person what you appreciate about them, or about life in general.

A Mother's Meditation on Gratitude

Set aside a quiet time during which you can reflect on some of the many things you could be thankful for. As a starting point, you could read the passage below to yourself or out loud, adapting it to your situation as you like.

There really is so much to be thankful for.

I am grateful for my children, for the delight and love they bring, for the sweet smell of their hair and the soft touch of their skin. For the first time they smiled at me or walked into my arms. For the meaning they bring to life. For receiving my love and lessons. For being themselves, for giving me their own love and lessons. Having them at all is a miracle, and the rest is details.

I appreciate myself. For the love I have given my children, all the diapers changed, all the dishes done. For the long hours I've worked, the hoops I've jumped through to keep all those balls up in the air. For the efforts I've made, the many times I've stayed patient, the many times I've found more inside to give when I thought I was empty. For all my sweating and suffering.

I appreciate my partner. For the ways he has loved me, the fun we've had together, the humor, and the companionship. For the times of support, understanding, and sympathy. For his sweating and suffering too.

I feel thankful for the life I've already had, for the good parts of my childhood, for everything I've learned, for good friends and beautiful sights. For the roof over my head and the bread on my table, for being able to have a life that is healthier, longer, and freer than most people have ever dreamed of. For this beautiful world, where each breath is a gift of air, each dawn a gift of light. For the plants and animals that die so I may live. For the extraordinary gift of evolution I carry in each cell of my body, for the capabilities accumulated during three and a half billion years of life's presence on our planet. For the wonder of the universe, for all the atoms in my body—the carbon in my bones, the oxygen and iron in my blood—that were born in the heart of an exploding star billions of years ago, to drift through space, to form a sun and planets, to form the hand that holds this book and the eye that reads this word. For all that was in order for me to be. For grace, for wisdom, for the sacred, for spirit as I know it. For this moment, this breath, this sight. For every good thing that was, that is, that ever will be.

> *It will be gone before you know it. The fingerprints on the wall appear higher and higher. Then suddenly they disappear.*
>
> Dorothy Evslin

Extremes of Mood

At one time or another, many mothers will experience forms of sadness that are so intense or chronic that they fall in the clinical range. Please see if any of the following descriptions apply to you, and if one does, you should consult with a professional right away.

- **Postpartum depression (PPD):** Depressed mood continuing past the "baby blues" (three to seven days postpartum) and lasting up to a year after childbirth; suffered by at least one in eight mothers. Often accompanied by severe anxiety or panic, spontaneous crying, agitation, insomnia, obsessional thoughts, lack of interest in the baby, or suicidal thinking. In the extreme, there may be psychotic delusions, often related to the baby. Making things worse, it is common to feel guilty about having depressed feelings at a time when a mother is "supposed" to be happy.

Good books and support organizations for PPD are listed in Appendix A. After an episode of PPD has seemed to resolve, there may still be an underlying disturbance in the endocrine system, or unstable or low mood; these should be considered with your doctor if you have ever had an episode of PPD.

- **Persistent depressive disorder:** Chronically low mood that occurs for most of the day, more days than not, for at least two years (but remember, you don't have to wait two years to seek help!). Some days can feel OK, but then the dark cloud descends again. It often coexists with anxiety, feelings of guilt or inadequacy, brooding about the past, or major depressive episodes.
- **Major depressive disorder:** Feelings of extreme sadness or despair lasting two weeks or longer, accompanied by hopelessness, fatigue, disturbed sleep or appetite, poor concentration, difficulty making decisions, feelings of worthlessness, withdrawal from family or friends, or suicidal thinking. When you add up the number of individuals who get depressed, the typical length of a depressive episode, and its impact on both functioning and experience of life, women worldwide are more burdened by depression than by any other health condition. About 10 percent of mothers are clinically depressed at any given time, and this rate jumps to 13 percent among women who have recently given birth. Of course, the percentage of mothers who will ever be clinically depressed is much higher, and the number of mothers who have depressed mood but do not meet the stringent criteria for clinical depression will be greater than those who are clinically depressed. Depression is best treated through the teamwork of:
  — *You:* Sometimes the first step is the hardest: admitting to yourself that you are, in fact, depressed. But once you

do, you can reach out to the things that will help you. Remember what worked the last time you were depressed; you probably found some things that helped, and there's a good chance they'll work this time too. Stick with it, and you will almost certainly feel better over time.

— *Your partner:* He can support you through understanding, extra help, affection, and encouragement. It might help him to read about depression in such books as *An Unquiet Mind* by Kay Redfield Jamison, MD, or *The Noonday Demon* by Andrew Solomon. He also needs to take extra care of himself in order to keep being supportive of you. It's also important to reach out to your friends.

— *A therapist:* There is more evidence that psychological factors cause depression than biochemical ones, and studies have shown that psychotherapy is as effective or better for many people than antidepressants (and without the side effects), plus generally more successful at preventing relapse. And a person can certainly take an antidepressant while going through therapy; a combination of treatment methods can sometimes be more effective than either one alone.

— *A physician:* Depression is a common complication of insomnia, chronic pain, illness, or medications (including oral contraceptives), and you should rule out these possibilities with your doctor. For the physiological treatment of depression, including antidepressants and herbs such as Saint-John's-wort, see chapter 5. In general, depression should be addressed through a combination of social support, stress reduction, optimizing physical health, psychotherapy, and—if necessary—medication.

- **Bipolar disorder:** Fundamental instability in mood, marked by at least one manic episode. Features of a manic episode include abnormally elevated or irritable mood, decreased need for sleep, grandiosity, distractibility, racing thoughts or speech, bursts of activity or agitation, or sudden shifts in mood (e.g., from euphoria to anger).

Bipolar disorder and major depression carry a serious risk of suicide. The death of a mother by her own hand is a devastating loss and lasting wound for her children, and there are *always* better options. Psychotherapy and medication are highly effective, plus people usually rally behind a mother when she lets them know she's really hit bottom. If you have been contemplating suicide, even abstractly (e.g., "the children would be better off if I were gone"), please immediately tell someone who cares about you as well as get professional help from a licensed therapist.

Key Ways to Turn Sadness into Contentment

- Take time to mourn the things you've lost since becoming a mom.
- Pay attention to the things that are going well.
- Talk back to helpless, pessimistic thoughts.
- Keep your sense of humor and perspective.
- Spend more time in sunlight.
- Make it a priority to get out and have some fun.
- Find support among friends.
- Take time to be grateful.
- Get professional help for depression or other mood disorders.

TURNING ANXIETY INTO SECURITY

> *We are, perhaps uniquely among the earth's creatures, the worrying animal. We worry away our lives, fearing the future, discontent with the present, unable to take in the idea of dying, unable to sit still.*
>
> Lewis Thomas

As a mother, you naturally have a sense of great responsibility for the life and well-being of your vulnerable child. But you are inherently unable to do much about many things that can affect him or her, such as diseases in other children, the safety of playground equipment, how other people drive, workplace policies, your partner's moods, or the conduct of childcare providers. No wonder you sometimes feel anxious!

Even seemingly small matters can have large stakes, as a single mother with a five-year-old son described: *When I dropped Kai off at soccer camp, I realized I'd forgotten his shoes. The coach said he couldn't play without them, so I left Kai there and raced off to get some shoes, with his parting words ringing in my ears: "This is the worst day of my life." Instead of driving 20 minutes each way to home and back, I figured it was best to try some stores nearby. But nothing was open because it was Saturday morning. I got so frustrated that I yelled at other cars, "Hurry up, move!" All the while I could see Kai standing alone on the sidelines, watching the other children, the minutes ticking by. I get so worried about letting him down: His dad has already done that big time, and I just can't stand the thought of me doing it too.*

Feelings of anxiety can also be triggered or increased by experiences you had as a child. For example, Rick worked with a mother whose son's fiery temperament was just like her dad's. Even though she knew intellectually that Liam was only a four-year-old, it made her body feel panicky whenever he got angry.

A heightened sense of vigilance after children is normal; it's Mother Nature's way of keeping your children safe from the local tiger. But anxiety that is over the top feels awful. It also wears on the body and mind, and it can lead people to be rigid, controlling, or overly cautious with their children. Let's explore some effective ways to feel more secure and less anxious.

Talking Back to Anxiety

It's really helpful to spotlight the inaccurate, illogical, or overly negative thoughts that make you anxious, and replace them with positive ones. By now, you're probably getting pretty good at this technique. Here are examples of the kinds of thoughts that tend to make mothers nervous, with some sample talk-back rebuttals.

- *Over-estimating the chances of a bad outcome*

NEGATIVE THOUGHT	POSITIVE ALTERNATIVES
He drives faster than me, so the baby is not safe in the car with him.	My husband drives no faster than most other people, and he has never been in a serious accident. He has driven many more miles than me; as a more experienced driver, it's OK for him to drive a little faster than me. We have a good car seat, and he is always careful to strap the baby in. He has promised to drive extra carefully with the baby in the car.

- *Assuming there's been a catastrophe*

NEGATIVE THOUGHT	POSITIVE ALTERNATIVES
They're late, they haven't called, something terrible has happened.	Maybe he was delayed getting Henry out of day care. They've been this late before. I know I tend to get worked up with worry, so I can't assume there is actually a real threat just because my body is panicky. Even if something terrible has actually happened, we'll get through it somehow.

- *Overgeneralizing*

NEGATIVE THOUGHT	POSITIVE ALTERNATIVES
Ava hangs back in kindergarten, so she won't have many friends growing up, and she'll be lonely all her life.	"Slow-to-warm" is a normal temperament. Ava is a normal five-year-old. There are lots of slow-to-warm people in the world, and many of them have happy lives and good friendships. There is no reason it can't be the same for Ava. Her teacher and I can probably help her find a friend in her class.

Retraining the Worry Impulse

Chronic worrying can become an almost automatic response to life, but the good news is you can retrain it. It just takes practice. Here are some of the best ways we know to get out of worry loops.

See sources of safety. Pay more attention to the reasons why you should feel safe, secure, and confident. You could make a mental list of the resources within you (intelligence, character, determination, good-heartedness) or in your environment (strong marriage, savings, friends). Notice how things usually work out alright; remind yourself that people who have been there for you in the past are likely to be there for you in the future too.

Be realistic. Try to think through whatever it is that you are worried about in a grounded, problem-solving sort of way. Ask yourself, *What's the chance of this actually happening?* Then figure out what you could do to prevent it or to cope with it if you had to.

Take action. Occasionally, worrying is just a disguised way to avoid acting. One mother was rueful as she admitted to Ricki: *I think I'm obsessing about the different ways to get Jamie to sleep through the night partly because I'm afraid to just pick one.* And sometimes we believe in a corner of the mind that worrying itself will ward off threats: *If I relax about the baby, that's when something awful will happen.*

But it's only real action that will solve the tangible problems that are making you anxious. Perhaps talk through your concerns with your partner or a friend and make a plan for what you'll actually do. Being active rather than passive will usually make you feel better.

Cultivate an attitude of acceptance. The painful truth is that many of the forces that will shape our precious children's lives are out of our hands, whether it's the temperament they were born with or the effects of thousands of interactions with other children. There's a peace in surrendering to this fact.

Don't overreact to your body. The brain draws conclusions about the world in part by reading the body's signals; in a sense, it reasons that "the world is scary because my body is nervous" rather than "my body is nervous because the world is scary." This kind of thinking helped keep our ancestors alive in the wild, but today it's like looking for road hazards by staring at the speedometer.

It's especially important for a mother to watch out for this tendency since depletion and stress make your body more reactive and "jumpy." Notice any inclination in yourself to be preoccupied with your body or hypersensitive to its sensations, and then put in a correction factor in the other direction, such as *I know I have a nervous stomach, so I need to remember that I should not assume that Ivy is really sick just because I feel queasy.*

Budget worry. Maybe it's reasonable to have the same thought ten times, but more than that is just too much. Instead, make an appointment with yourself to worry. For example, it could be an hour from now. If an alarming thought arises before then, tell yourself that you'll be open for business in just a few minutes, but right now the person who staffs the worry window is on her break. Or pick a specific period, say for 20 minutes each morning, when you will worry about a particular issue. Keep to that schedule and try to worry hard within it. For the rest of the time, tell your anxious thoughts that you will give them your full attention soon, but only during their regular appointment.

Derail your train of (anxious) thought. Our worries often have a mechanical, repetitive quality, like a train doing laps around a track. There are a number of ways to stop them, such as thinking about something that requires concentration like counting down from one hundred by sevens, or repeatedly reciting a prayer or mantra. You can distract yourself in good ways such as making cookies with your toddler, playing a sport, or reading a novel (with a happy ending!). Simply focusing for a minute or two on some aspect of your environment, such as the grain on a wooden table or the steam coming off a cup of tea, is usually calming. Or you could meditate (see page 66), which has been shown to be quite effective in lowering anxiety. (If worrying keeps you awake at night, please see our suggestions about sleep in chapter 4.)

Settle your body. Breathing techniques (see page 51), massage, or simply a hot shower can reduce anxiety and lift your overall mood. Cutting down on caffeine or eliminating it entirely can also make a difference. Instead of coffee, try some soothing herbal teas such as chamomile or peppermint.

Talk it out. When you tell someone about your concerns, you get them out of your head and into the open where you and the other person can consider how serious they actually are. It'll make you feel better to hear that others have similar fears, and you can also find out how they dealt with them.

Avoid "doom scrolling." Consider how your information diet affects your mood. News feeds and social media can amplify anxiety through comparison, alarm, and overload—especially when you're already depleted. If you find yourself spiraling into late-night scrolling or asking AI for reassurance, treat that as a sign to come back to your body and to real-world support.

> *Motherhood brings as much joy as ever, but it still brings boredom, exhaustion, and sorrow, too. Nothing else ever will make you as happy or as sad, as proud or as tired, for nothing is quite as hard as helping a person develop his own individuality—especially while you struggle to keep your own.*
>
> Marguerite Kelly and Ella Parsons

Dealing with Traumatic Stress

Lots of things with children will give your nervous system a jolt: a sudden yelp of pain from the other room, an unexpected call from the preschool director, or a dog on the sidewalk lunging at your stroller. After a few minutes, the fright wears off, and everything settles back down to normal. But sometimes the shock of an event, or series of related events, is so great as to be truly traumatic. For example, studies have found that mothers whose children have had serious illnesses or traumatic experiences themselves often experience intrusive and intense images or memories, problems concentrating or making decisions, a heightened reactivity, or physical symptoms such as a pounding heart or headaches.

Other stressors can also have traumatic effects, as one mother described: *Paul and I got a babysitter for our first night out since Jayden was born. I went over all the instructions and gave her the phone number for the restaurant. When we got home, we heard the baby crying and crying. The babysitter said he woke up soon after we left and had been crying since, nearly two hours! Incredibly, she hadn't thought she should call us. I rushed upstairs and finally settled Jayden, but I felt terrible. Since then, I haven't been able to leave him with anyone but Paul. It makes me feel trapped in my house, but I don't care, I can't let it happen again.*

Additionally, if you've ever experienced trauma that is not directly related to child-rearing—such as abuse as a child, sexual assault as an adult, or spousal abuse*—that can cast a shadow over your life as a

---

* It is estimated that in the US, 1 in 4 girls have been sexually molested, 1 in 4 women will be the victim of attempted or completed sexual assault, and 41 percent will be the victim of intimate partner violence. (Note that these estimates can vary because of the groups studied and the definitions used by researchers.)

mother. For example, putting your child in a setting that's like the one in which you were traumatized, such as being left alone with a male caregiver, might make your heart pound. Trauma can also be vicarious, especially if you witnessed it as an impressionable child. One of Rick's clients saw years of loud, drunken fights between her parents, one of which put her mother in the hospital. She said, *When my kids yell at each other, I feel frozen inside and far away. That's when it's really hard to just be a mom.*

If traumatic stress is affecting you, here are some ways to help yourself cope:

- *Really acknowledge the intensity and seriousness of what happened*, rather than telling yourself that you are weak or flawed to have let it get to you.
- *Share your experience with others* who care about you. Besides helping you feel better, research has found that talking about a traumatic experience can strengthen your immune system.
- *Consider joining a support group,* such as one for adults who were abused as children, or for parents of children with serious illnesses.
- *Take extra care of yourself,* with good meals, plenty of rest, and time to relax. Try to maintain familiar routines as much as you can.
- *Seek professional help* if you feel panicky, troubled by intrusive thoughts or images, or unable to continue functioning in your job or family. Both counseling and medication have been shown to be quite successful with traumatic stress and other forms of anxiety.

Key Ways to Turn Fear into Security

- Replace anxious thoughts with realistic and hopeful ones.
- Retrain the worry impulse.
- Take action to change the things that concern you.
- Routinely relax your body.
- Get professional help for chronic anxiety or experiences of traumatic stress.

TURNING SHAME INTO A SENSE OF WORTH

It's easy to feel like you're falling short. Your kids probably think that you are the solution to every problem. There's more work to do in a day than anyone could possibly finish. Few of the people in the different parts of your life—home, work, friends, your own parents or siblings—are really aware of the juggling you've got to do in the other ones, so it's hard for them to be understanding when you can't keep every single ball in the air. It's easy to think that your children reflect on you, as a mother related to Rick: *We were sitting in the pediatrician's waiting room, my baby started to cry and I couldn't settle her down. I caught looks from other mothers that made me feel I was doing everything wrong.*

These seeds of shame find fertile soil in the minds of many mothers. Because girls and women are bombarded with messages that equate appearance and worth, the weight gain and other bodily changes that are almost universal after having babies can lower your self-esteem. And motherhood can be isolating, further eroding the sense of worth that in the past was refueled through social connections. One mother told Jan: *Now I spend many hours each day with no one to talk to besides my baby. Before, there were lots of people to joke or talk with at the office, and just doing that reminded me in lots of little ways that I was making a difference.* Girls and women get many messages to put the wants of others first; it is a short step from "my wants don't matter" to "my self doesn't matter."

Plus, there could be personality characteristics that make a person extra vulnerable to the challenges to self-worth that come with children. Do any of these apply to you?

- You set high standards for yourself.
- You are easily embarrassed or even humiliated by criticism.
- You depend on approval from others for a sense of worth.
- As a child, you received frequent criticism from parents, coaches, teachers, siblings, or other kids.
- You have a relentless inner critic.

For any one of these various reasons, it's understandable if you occasionally feel embarrassed, self-critical, inadequate, guilty, or remorseful. A bit of this is inevitable in any parent with a conscience, since raising kids is such a complicated and difficult business that everyone blows it some of the time. But if you're feeling guilt or shame that's *undeserved*, it's no good for either you or your children. Getting unfairly critical or angry with yourself worsens your well-being, makes it harder to cope, and leaves a bruised sadness inside. Therefore, it's really important to feel as good about yourself as you truly deserve.

Talking Back to Shame

If you berate yourself for being less than a perfect mother, think about what you would do if you heard another person speaking to a friend—or your child!—the way you speak to yourself. Surely you would stick up for your friend or your child; why not yourself? Here are a few examples:

- *Linking your worth to your child's behavior*

NEGATIVE THOUGHT	POSITIVE ALTERNATIVES
My first-grader, Mark, is misbehaving and people are staring. I'm a klutz as a mother.	Mark is out of line but I am not. I am not Mark. Most people understand that kids from good parents sometimes misbehave. People who know me think I'm a good parent. If strangers come to a snap judgment about me, that's their problem.

- *Comparing yourself to your mother*

NEGATIVE THOUGHT	POSITIVE ALTERNATIVES
I'm just not handling things as well as my mom did.	My memories of my mother are those of a child, with little real idea of what she was thinking or the mistakes that occurred out of my sight. I probably look pretty good to my kids too. She received more support than I have gotten from her neighbors, relatives, and community. She felt safe with us playing outside, and she didn't have to drive us everywhere. Considering what I have to deal with, I am actually doing very well.

- *Feeling bad about being needy*

NEGATIVE THOUGHT	POSITIVE ALTERNATIVES
I need so much from my partner and family. It's shameful that I can't manage on my own.	Mothers throughout history have always relied on tremendous support from others. That's the normal state of affairs, and that's what my child needs me to have. There's an idea in our culture that everyone is supposed to be super self-reliant. Most other societies emphasize community much more than we do. While I do get some help, the truth is that I handle almost everything on my own.

- *Equating your fundamental value as a human being to your performance as a parent*

NEGATIVE THOUGHT	POSITIVE ALTERNATIVES
I yelled at Mateo during his tantrum, and I feel like a bad person.	What I do is not who I am. I blew it for about 30 seconds. That's a tiny fraction of a life. And the part of me that came out then is just a small aspect of my total personality. With Mateo, I can repair what happened. He loves me, and he knows that I love him.

Forgiving Yourself

We all make mistakes. And the more complicated, ambiguous, and changeable the task—in other words, the more it resembles motherhood—the more mistakes we are bound to make. Most of them are little ones: forgetting to bring along snacks for a walk in the park, missing a meeting at the preschool, leaving a baby in a wet diaper too long. But there isn't a parent alive who hasn't blown it big time with a child one way or another, whether screaming and yelling, missing an obvious safety hazard, or simply being too busy to really pay attention.

One of the hardest parts of raising children is watching ourselves make the same mistake over and over. It seems unforgivable! But it takes time to change. There are four stages in any kind of learning or personal growth, and we need to be easy on ourselves in the process. Let's suppose you've been snapping too harshly at your kids:

Stage 1. Unconscious incompetence: You're not aware that there's a problem.

Stage 2. Conscious incompetence: You realize you shouldn't be doing it, but you just can't stop yourself. This is the most uncomfortable stage.

Stage 3. Conscious competence: The inclination to snap harshly still arises within your mind, but you catch it and do something different, such as take a big breath and speak more calmly.

Stage 4. Unconscious competence: The tendency doesn't even arise. Sometimes it's hard to remember that you used to act in a different way.

The fact that change takes a while doesn't make you a bad parent. Errors come with the territory of raising a family, they are unavoidable, you are trying to correct them, and you deserve to be forgiven for them. If something is bothering you, you could talk about it with someone who knows you well as a mother, such as your partner, good friend, or your own mom, and then ask that person for forgiveness. You can also forgive yourself, using the steps of self-forgiveness in the box.

Steps of Self-Forgiveness

1. Name the thing that you feel guilty or ashamed about.
2. Reflect on the total situation, including your part in it, and sort out in your mind what you feel rightfully responsible for and what you do not. Separate out the rest as bad luck, beyond anyone's reasonable control, or the responsibility of others. Regret may be warranted for those pieces of the puzzle, but not remorse.
3. Really let yourself take personal responsibility for the parts that are appropriate. Notice any emotions that come with the sense of responsibility, such as sadness, relief, guilt, embarrassment, or shame. Let yourself truly feel them for a bit. When it seems right, let them go, using the techniques you've learned.
4. Resolve to yourself what you will do about the parts you are responsible for. Sincerely decide how you will acknowledge your responsibility to others, make amends, or act differently in the future.
5. Now, let in a sense of forgiveness for yourself. You've taken responsibility for your part, you've felt bad about it, you've figured out what you can do, and it's alright to move on. In your mind, you can tell yourself things like *I am forgiven for ______*, or *You are forgiven for ______*, or *I forgive myself for ______*. You could imagine your children or partner forgiving you. You might imagine that

a nurturing being of great integrity—perhaps a specific person such as your own mother or a kind of guardian angel—understands everything that has happened and forgives you completely. Or, if this is meaningful to you, you could ask for God's forgiveness and allow that grace to fill your heart.

Nurturing Your Sense of Worth

Things that might make you feel guilty or inadequate—from frustrating struggles with a child to critical looks from other parents—can happen at any time, so it's important to nourish your sense of worth on a regular basis. Here are some good ways to do this.

Carry a picture of yourself as a child. You probably have pictures of your children on your phone and take them with you wherever you go, and one look is all it takes to feel warmth and love. But you were once such a little person yourself, and within you today is still a precious being that deserves to be treated with love and respect. One of the best and simplest ways we know to keep that feeling alive—of your innate worth and the need to nurture yourself—is to find a picture of when you were a baby or young child and carry it with you. You might put it in front of the driver's license in your wallet. Each time you reach for some cash or a credit card, that innocent little face will remind you that you are the same dear person, just older and more seasoned by life.

Appreciate your accomplishments. As you go along, try to pay conscious attention to the things you get done. In a typical day, you could keep a running list of all the tasks you've completed, down to the details. Review it in the evening, maybe with your partner, to see the incredible number of things you accomplish each day.

Take some credit for how great your children are doing. Unless something is terribly wrong, your children are thriving, and you have had a lot to do with that. From time to time, take a few minutes to reflect on the many ways you have nurtured and guided them.

Pay attention to positive feedback. Probably many times each day, your children, mate, coworkers, or friends pay you a compliment, appreciate your work, give you affection, or let you know they like you. It could be obvious—a child running to give you a hug—or implicit, like being asked to be copresident of your mothers' club. But in either case, it is sincere and real, and you can take it in.

Ask for acknowledgment. This may seem a little bold, but there is no law against asking for legitimate recognition, appreciation, or praise. You could take the plunge with your partner or a friend and just ask for some positive feedback about how you are doing as a mother, or about yourself in general. Or, if you're paid a compliment, say thanks and then ask if the person might be able to explain a bit why he or she sees you that way.

Reflect on your fundamental worth as a person. Take a minute or more every day as a small sanctuary in which you focus on the goodness inside you. You may also try some of the meditations on worth that are listed in the box.

Meditations on Your Worth

You can do the mini meditations below separately or in combination. Just find a place where you can be quiet for a few minutes, close your eyes, and begin.

- Think back over the last hour and recall as many things as you can that you accomplished. Think back over the past day and recall some ways you held your temper, had patience, were determined, or otherwise showed good character.

- Imagine how much you matter to your children. Think about the many ways they depend on you. If you went out of town for a week, what would be missing in their lives?
- Visualize one or more people who care about, like, and respect you. Take a moment to imagine each person speaking from his or her heart about your good qualities. Let it really sink in that you are seen and accepted, wanted and cherished.
- See if you can experience a sense of connection with these people or others. You could feel this in your body, or visualize lines of energy linking you together, or have an intuition of the philosophical and scientific truth that all seemingly separate things blend into and depend on each other. If you can, let that experience of connection extend from these individuals to other people, perhaps to the entire human race. Try to sense that you belong to that larger family. Finally, see if you can shift from looking outward at all these people to taking their perspective and seeing that they all have a connection with *you*.
- Imagine your connections with other moms, starting with those closest to you and extending ultimately to all mothers alive today. Feel how you are joined to these women by shared experiences and commitments. It is an honorable community, the wellspring of humanity, and you are a valued member.
- Let an awareness grow of your innermost being, inherently good and wise, your essential self. Nothing can taint

that inner being or alter its quality. Let a sense of its worth fill you. In the deepest sense possible, who you *are* is that being, and its worth is your worth.

Sticking Up for Yourself with Others

One mother of a bouncy two-year-old told Rick this story: *We were houseguests with my husband's best friend, his wife, and their three children. Their home is very nice, with lots of expensive bric-a-brac. I was a nervous wreck, keeping Lily out of trouble. The wife kept making little comments, always with this sweet smile, about ways she disciplined her own children. By the end of the weekend, I was ready to wring her neck.*

For some reason, all sorts of people—perfect strangers, nonparents, perhaps your mother-in-law—feel entitled to comment freely about how a woman could do a better job as a mother, yet they wouldn't dream of giving the same level of advice to a shopkeeper, plumber, architect—or father. There's a place for gentle suggestions if they're welcome, but unwanted advice contains the implicit message that whatever you are doing is wrong. That message comes through in other ways as well: nasty looks from other people, criticisms from relatives, comparisons to other parents, and so on. Besides being embarrassing, these comments can prey on your mind, breeding self-doubt and a sense of inadequacy. Here are some useful strategies for dealing with them:

- Anticipate situations that are likely to generate judgments about you or your children. For instance, maybe it's wiser to leave the kids home with a sitter when you go out to dinner with your husband's parents.
- Brush off a comment with one of your own, such as *Yes, there are lots of ways to be a good parent.*

- Take pressure off yourself by postponing judgment about what was said. Later on, within your own mind or by talking with a friend, you can see if there is any wheat amid the chaff.
- Ask your partner to stick up for you (if that's a problem, see chapters 6, 7, and 8).
- Confront the comment directly. You can address the values that underlie it by asserting your own, as in *Actually, John and I think it's more important for a child to feel loved than to have good manners.* You can back up your views with scientific research, such as *No, many studies have shown that going to babies when they cry helps make them more secure and confident when they're older.* If you have to, you can go right to the heart of the matter: *Mom, you did the best you could and I love you a ton. But, in some ways, I've decided to raise Amy differently.*
- Tell the person commenting that you would rather not hear any feedback or advice unless you specifically ask for it.
- Remind yourself of several specific ways you are clearly a good mother.

Treating Yourself Well

We know many mothers who dote on their children and are loving with their partner but have a really hard time doing anything nice for themselves. For instance, Sasha, a mother of three, had worked nearly full-time throughout her kids' early years for a number of catering companies on an as-needed basis. When her youngest was still in preschool, the economy had a downturn and catering work dried up. She and her husband decided that she should not look for work for six months and be a full-time homemaker instead. She told Rick: *Even though I'm home, I still always have to be doing something. I make lists and check things off: Fold the laundry, call the dentist, get some milk. I feel totally guilty if I'm just sitting, even for a few minutes. I can't relax and read a magazine or call a friend. If I did, I'd feel like a goof-off.* Jenny laughed at herself in Jan's office while telling a similar story: *I love a sale, and I always get the kids stuff they don't really need. But I cannot bring myself to buy a new pair of loafers to replace the funky ones I've had for five years.*

Do you find it hard to do nice things for yourself? If so, we suggest you experiment with deliberately going against the grain. For example, buy a bottle of luxury shampoo instead of your usual, more sensible brand. Try taking a longer but more interesting way home from work, even if that means dinner will be 15 minutes later. Or get your partner to watch the kids on Saturday morning while you take a long bath.

Key Ways to Turn Shame into Self-Worth

- Understand the psychological factors within you that make you prone to feeling inadequate; try to get some distance from them and even let them go.
- Stick up *for* yourself *to* yourself (e.g., talk back to shame).
- Actively forgive yourself for being human and imperfect, and for not changing overnight.
- Carry a picture of yourself as a child.
- Notice all the things you get done each day.
- Reflect on how well your children are doing—and take some credit for that.
- Allow yourself to take in positive feedback.
- Stick up for yourself with others.
- Do some nice things for yourself.

TURNING ANGER INTO A PEACEFUL HEART

Elaine had three children ages two, four, and seven, and she worked full-time as a computer programmer for a large brokerage company. She had been meeting weekly with Rick for several months, talking about her marriage with Dennis, before she felt comfortable enough to tell her deepest, darkest secret. Normally self-controlled and forthright, her voice was sad and hesitant: *Sometimes I get pretty mad at my kids. Like yesterday morning. I was making lunches for day care, and running late. I heard Leo and Noah begin screaming at each other. Dennis had already taken Ariana to school, so I went into the living room and they were fighting over some stupid toy. Leo shoved his little brother and he fell and hit his head on the floor. I picked Noah up and just started yelling at Leo. He looked scared but I kept yelling anyway. I was so tired of him pushing his brother around. He started crying and I stopped yelling. I got a little calmer and we talked about what had happened and how he couldn't hit or shove his brother. It was OK, but I felt upset for a long time afterwards. The person I was most mad at for the rest of the day was me.*

Let's be realistic: It's completely normal to get angry with your children. Or with your partner, the in-laws, a friend—or yourself. Studies have found that the more children a woman has, the more time she spends with them or doing housework, and the more hassles she has with childcare or her kids, the more angry she's likely to be. There's no need to feel guilty about anger itself. The real question is, what can you do about it?

On the one hand, anger is a healthy emotion. It shines a bright light on things that should be different—like a child's incessant whining, a partner's broken promises, or some stupid workplace policy that keeps you from your kids—and energizes you to try to change them. Bottling up anger numbs your other feelings as well, and it wears on your health.

Acting like you are not mad when you really are is inauthentic and teaches kids to put on a false face themselves—not a good lesson.

On the other hand, anger takes you on an emotional roller coaster that stresses your body and can leave you feeling bad for hours. And no other emotion has such an impact on relationships. When Mom or Dad gets mad, that's scary and often overwhelming for kids since their parents are so much bigger, have tremendous power, and are so important. In a marriage, frequent anger is very wounding; after a while, anyone would start wanting to step back from a person who's mad a lot of the time. There's a saying that getting angry with someone is like throwing hot coals with bare hands: Both people get burned.

Fortunately, there's a healthy middle path between tight-lipped self-censoring and boiling-over rage. In this section, we'll be looking at a number of ways to work with anger wisely, inside your own mind. (Chapters 6, 7, and 8 address anger in an intimate relationship.)

Stop Things from Building Up

We usually get mad in two stages. First there's the priming: tension, frustration, bodily discomfort, fatigue, gripes, etc. mount up like a growing pile of dynamite. Then comes the firecracker that sets it all off: *I got home from a hard day at work, the little one was getting a cold, her big brother was whiny and clingy, and the phone kept ringing. Then the garbage disposal stopped working and the sink wouldn't empty. That was the last straw. It's stupid, but I jabbed the drain over and over with the end of a wooden spoon, I was so mad!*

During the priming phase, try to defuse things *before* there's a blowup. Here are a few ideas.

Don't overgive. For example, don't agree to chair the annual fundraiser at the preschool when you don't really want to—and then resent it later. One trick is to imagine asking your future self, the one who will be stuck with the work, how she will feel and what she would like you to do. Another is to adopt the blanket policy of never agreeing to anything until you've had some time to think it over.

Blow off steam as you go along. Try not to accumulate residues of irritation from individual interactions. Let's say you've just had the usual struggle to get your toddler to eat something. Before shifting gears into the next thing, you could wash your face with warm water, do something loud and goofy with your child, or shake your arms and exhale vigorously.

Take a break before you get to the breaking point. Most parents become quite frayed by the time they've been alone with a young child for three or four hours. Make it a serious priority to find some way—*any* way—to give yourself a break before your pot boils over. Maybe you need to arrange a regular get-together with another mom, go out to a setting with other children like a park, schedule an hour or so of childcare in the middle of the day, or give your child screen time for half an hour.

Understand What's Making You Angry

When you're mad, there's typically more to the story than just anger. Let's say you've had a long day on your job and now you're in the grocery store with your three-year-old son, and all you want to do is get home, make some dinner, and relax. But he wants some candy, you say no, and he throws a major tantrum. People are staring, you feel mortified, somehow you get him out of the store and into your car, and then you really yell at him. In that moment, the intensity of your anger is at least a six or seven on a ten-point scale.

But now let's change some of the elements of the situation. Suppose it's a Saturday morning instead and you're feeling rested and relaxed. How intense do you think your anger would be in that case? Probably less: maybe one to three on the anger scale. Or suppose that you're at home, not out at the store, when he throws his tantrum; no one is watching you, and you don't have to care what anyone is thinking. How angry do you think you'd be then? Again, probably less. Fatigue and embarrassment amplified your feelings by five or so "points" that had nothing to do with the actual seriousness of your son's misbehavior. And when you understand this, suddenly you're a lot less mad.

Sorting out the various factors involved lets you see how much a situation is actually worth getting mad about. If it's really just a "one" or a "two," feeling any angrier than that is needless aggravation. This sorting also helps you protect your child or partner from getting blasted about things that really don't have anything to do with them: It's not their fault that your boss is a pain in the neck or the commute was awful today or you got stuck at the house waiting for a plumber who never showed up.

Let's see how to deal with common factors that add topspin to a mother's anger.

If you think your child is deliberately manipulating you. Manipulation involves deception, and most children below the age of seven or so have not yet developed the cognitive abilities required to be deliberately tricky. Your child just wants what he wants, and you happen to be in the way. As a normal developmental process, he needs to try different ways of getting what he wants in order to find out what works. When you hold your ground and say no, he receives a little lesson that he needs to find a different want, or a better way of getting it. Of course, it could take dozens or even hundreds of repetitions before the lesson sinks in; it could certainly feel frustrating, but it's not manipulation.

If you see something in your child that you don't like in yourself. One of Rick's clients, Wanda, had grown up in a strict and traditional home, and she was always getting into trouble as a little girl for her tomboy ways. Over time, she learned to push down her more aggressive and independent parts and act like a highly "feminine" girl. Then, years later, she had a daughter herself. To her dismay, Emma wanted to run around with the boys, yelling and building forts and sword fighting. She was blunt and outspoken with other kids, and had no interest in acting nicey-nicey just to get along. Wanda often felt embarrassed by her daughter. She told Rick: *Part of me is rooting for Emma, but another part thinks that girls should not act like that. I keep waiting for some big punishment to come down on her, like people yelling at her. Even though it never happens, I keep feeling nervous. So I'm always after her to be different. It's like* I'm *afraid of getting punished when she acts that way.*

By becoming more aware of the sources of her reactions to Emma, Wanda was able to see her as simply a bright, lively, and lovable child without the added layer of being upset about her daughter's so-called tomboyishness. She also remembered that it had upset her to have grown-ups angry with her when she was a kid, so it wasn't going to be any good for Emma either. If Emma was ever actually too pushy or too wild, what worked for Wanda was compassionate firmness, saturated in love for the wonderful qualities in her high-spirited daughter.

If you're prickly about any challenge to your authority. You are the ultimate authority until your children are 18, and they need to know that. If you feel confident and matter-of-fact about your authority, you'll usually be able to exercise it without having to make a big deal about it. It sounds backwards, but reminding yourself deep down that you have much more power than your child, and that you have plenty of ways to make it stick, makes it less necessary for you to prove it. It's also normal for kids to challenge their parents from time to time in order to clarify where the limits are. Excess anger on a parent's part about that natural process slows down a child's learning, and it could in fact lead to an older child or adolescent becoming oppositional.

If your partner is a lightning rod for your irritation with the kids. You could let him know that you're venting about the children, and not angry with him personally. And you can deal with your irritation with the kids directly, by doing what's possible to change things so they're less grating on you.

If your kids are a lightning rod for your irritation with your partner. Merely becoming aware of this usually makes it stop since it's about the last thing most parents would ever want to do. And it's a wake-up call to address issues directly with your partner.

If issues with your job are spilling over onto your family. Take a look at pages 381 to 387 in chapter 9.

If your own childhood is getting mixed into your anger. Like getting really mad at one child picking on another, because that's what happened to *you*. Or becoming tense at meals because your dad would usually be drinking by then when you were a kid, and he could fly off the handle. Simply recognizing childhood issues transferred into the present can start you on a path of separating them from the here-and-now realities of your life. Then you can work with them in their own right—including with the ideas and tools in this book.

If you're taking things too personally. Young children generally have no idea of their impact on their mom and dad. It's not realistic to expect the same empathy or consideration for yourself from your child that you would from another adult. Kids are like a force of nature; it's not *personal* when a bull knocks over crystal in a china shop.

And it's not just your kids. The intentions we attribute to others make a big difference in how we feel. Consider this adaptation of an ancient parable: *Imagine you are sitting on a boat on a river in the fog. Suddenly there is a loud crash against your boat and you are tipped over into the cold water. You come up sputtering and see that another boat full of laughing people has intentionally run into you; how do you feel? Now imagine the same situation, the same crash and dunking, but this time you come up sputtering and see that a submerged log has drifted into your boat; how do you feel?*

For better or worse, the world is basically one log after another—whether it's your son's snit fit, policies at the preschool, or your boss's latest brainstorm—and most of it is not about you personally. Even reactions that seem to be about you, such as a partner's criticism, were set in motion long ago, shaped by a biology, culture, and individual history that have nothing to do with you. Nobody likes getting whacked by "logs," and of course it makes sense to manage them as skillfully as possible. But if you can treat them more like impersonal facts, they won't make you as angry.

If you feel frustrated. Parts of parenthood are inherently frustrating, and frustration is a major trigger for anger. For example, there's no way anyone could possibly do everything on your daily to-do list in just one day, the needs of home and work pull in opposite directions, and you can't *make* your partner see it your way if he genuinely disagrees. All completely normal—and normally aggravating. One way to cope is to admit to yourself, and perhaps to others, that you cannot change certain situations: You accept things as they are and surrender to the way it is. Doing so usually brings a kind of peace. It also sends a healthy message that you can't do it all, and you shouldn't have to try. And it sometimes influences other people such as your partner to help out more.

Another way to cope with frustration is to lower your standards. For example, if you become more willing for your son to wear yesterday's grass-stained overalls, you'll feel less pressured about doing the laundry. You could also focus your attention on what you are doing or could be doing to improve the situation rather than on the places where you're being stymied. Or think about the future: Most things involving children really do get better over time.

Put On the Brakes

If you've ever yelled at your child in anger, you know that sick feeling you get later, after you've calmed down and started thinking about what had happened. Instead, walk away from the situation, put yourself in a time-out, yell into a towel or pillow, or call your partner or a friend. If you still have trouble controlling yourself, you're not alone. Most counties have anonymous text, phone, or chat-based support lines running 24 hours a day for parents to blow off steam and get practical ideas about child-rearing. These hotlines can also refer a mom to support groups or other community resources, such as low-fee childcare.

In less extreme situations, you might like to consider taking up the practice, for a day or longer, of not speaking to your children in an angry way. We are definitely not suggesting that you suppress your emotions, but rather that you:

- Sense down to the more vulnerable feelings—like fear, hurt, or disappointment—that usually lie beneath anger, and focus your awareness on them.
- Express whatever might be appropriate to your children about these softer feelings by saying things like: *I feel really scared when you run ahead at the mall, like something bad might happen to you, and to me that would be the worst thing in the world.* Or *I feel hurt and sad when you scream at me.*
- Do whatever you need to do in the way of correcting, reprimanding, or disciplining your child, but without losing your temper.

If you like, you can adapt this approach to your partner as well. No matter who you use it with, this practice helps you become more aware of the deeper feelings beneath anger, and more comfortable and skillful at expressing them. Then it will also be easier for a child—or your partner—to hear what you have to say.

This does not mean that you should turn anger toward others against yourself. Some mothers yell at themselves in their head, or even out loud. Some go further, pulling out their hair, abusing laxatives, or hitting or cutting themselves. If you ever do that sort of thing, please know that you are far from alone. Millions of other women have had similar issues, and feeling angry with yourself or ashamed for doing it just adds to the problem. As a first step, you should tell someone such as a close friend, your partner, a parent or relative, or a counselor on a telephone hotline. After that, please contact a therapist and get some professional help. The person in the world who least deserves your punishment is *yourself.*

Ask Your Heart

A client of Rick's told this story: *I was arguing with my husband about going back to work and he wanted me to stay home. I was getting madder and madder, but something else was happening too. It was like a part of me was watching the whole thing very calmly. After a while, I ran out of steam, and for a minute there was just that calmness. Then I did something I'd never done before. In a way, I asked the calmness for what it thought. Immediately, there was the sense of an answer, that the right approach was to be strong and confident and just go forward with what I knew to be right without quarreling about it, just start looking for work with self-respect and see what I found and then make my decision based on what was real. I didn't just hear how I needed to be, I* felt *that way. He asked what I was thinking and I told him, while I was feeling strong and confident, kind of dignified. He grumbled a little but didn't blow up again, and he seemed to accept more what I was saying. I spent about a month looking around for work. Once in a while, I'd think back to the experience and feel that sense of strength and confidence again. I found a pretty good job and we talked about it. It felt right to me, and he got some of that feeling too. I took it and I've been really happy that I did.*

Anger is like a storm at sea. On the surface, waves are roiling and spray is flying. But deeper down, it's much calmer. At almost any moment when you're angry, you can look down there for wisdom and guidance. To make those depths more real to yourself, ask your heart what might be a better way to handle the situation that's making you angry. You could put your awareness into the area of your heart and imagine asking a specific question—*What should I say? What matters most? What does she really need here? What would be best for everyone?*—or simply be open to your heart's perspective. Let both the meaning and the feeling of the answer fill you, pushing the surface froth of anger to the margins of your mind.

Key Ways to Turn Anger into Peace

- Don't let things build up, don't overgive, and blow off steam as you go along.
- Recognize beliefs or perspectives that are turbocharging your anger.
- Try to sense down to the softer emotions beneath anger, like hurt or fear; acknowledge those to yourself or express them to others.
- If you feel like you're going to blow up, walk away or call a friend.
- Get professional help if you are directing anger at yourself in harmful ways.
- Ask your heart for guidance.

✧ ✧ ✧

With the rush of changes and responsibilities in your life, it's no wonder you have some intense emotional responses. Sadness, anxiety, shame, anger: These come with the territory of deep caring for your family, but with some sustained effort, you can usually keep them from overwhelming you. There is so much you can handle by reaching in for the strength that resides within you, and by reaching out for the support of others who care about you and your children.

PART THREE

Nurturing Your Body

It's so important to tend to your physical health. But taking care of yourself could feel like adding yet more things to an already very long to-do list. With everything else clamoring for your time and attention, it's all too easy to push aside the actions that would add up to long-term wellness. That's why the next two chapters give you lots of options, so you can pick the ones that are the simplest to fit into your daily life.

Chapter 4 focuses on prevention, on commonsense practices—such as more sleep or better nutrition—that will keep you feeling well. Chapter 5 addresses what to do if you're already getting depleted, including many ways to replenish and balance your gastrointestinal, nervous, endocrine, and immune systems.

If it seems like your health has started to head downhill right in the middle of trying to raise a family, that can feel pretty scary. Your support may not be the greatest, and now your body is letting you down too. Thankfully, there is a lot you can do to nourish and settle the very roots of your body, to prevent and to heal the drainage and dysregulation of depletion.

CHAPTER FOUR

Staying Well

Alana, a 33-year-old real estate agent with two daughters aged six and two, came to Ricki for her annual gynecological visit. Alana showed off pictures of her children, whose red hair matched her husband's, and she laughed softly as she added, *They've got his feistiness too.* Before doing the exam, Ricki asked how she was feeling, and she said, *Fine, I guess.* Alana paused, and Ricki could tell that she didn't want to seem like she was complaining or unable to cope, so she told Alana that raising her own young daughter had worn her out more than a 100-hour-per-week obstetrics residency. *Yes,* Alana replied. *It's just been very physically taxing, like running myself to the ground, pushing my body to the edge of its capacity. For example, I hardly notice what I eat but I'm really careful about the girls. I stay up late to pay bills or just relax since it's the only time, but then it all starts again early the next morning. It's all making me feel more and more run down.*

Ricki nodded in understanding, having heard essentially the same story literally thousands of times before: a dedicated mom working harder than she ever has, with less time than ever to eat well or sleep or exercise, letting her own needs fall to the lowest priority. On most days, Alana was taking out more from her body's reserves than she was putting back in, so she was becoming gradually more depleted.

No one wants her experience of raising children to be shadowed by fatigue, nagging aches and pains, or emerging health problems. Not only is it a shame, it's also harder to function at a high level at home, at work, or in a relationship when you're running yourself into the ground. Many mothers have more or less resigned themselves to this condition, but the fact is that with only a few changes, most moms can be just as healthy after kids as they were before. The mothers we know who stay energetic, avoid illness, and keep some reserves in their "health bank" do these essential things:

- Get enough sleep.
- Eat right.
- Exercise regularly.
- Keep a basic balance in their lives.
- Have regular checkups.

This chapter is like a road map plus operating manual for your body, with many practical details. If a topic doesn't apply to you, just skip ahead to the next section.

> *Health is a state of complete physical, mental, and social well-being and not merely the absence of disease or infirmity.*
>
> Platform for Action of the Fourth World Conference on Women

GETTING ENOUGH SLEEP

There's an old saying: *The journey of a thousand miles begins with the first step, and the journey to health starts with sleep.* Most people need about eight hours of sleep each day; a person with a hardworking, stressful life—like a mother—usually needs even more, and it is vital to make sure you're getting enough. Insufficient sleep can lead to gastrointestinal troubles, a weakened immune system, and slow repair of strained or sore muscles acquired through routine activities like hauling children out of car seats. It also causes poor concentration and memory, lowers mood, and shortens a person's fuse.

When Your Children Are Little

> *There was never a child so lovely but his mother was glad to get him asleep.*
>
> Ralph Waldo Emerson

If you've got a baby or toddler, these steps should help you get more sleep. Some of them involve an active partner in parenting (for simplicity, we'll refer to a father); if you don't have that partner, there are other suggestions here that still should be useful for you.

Ask Dad. There's no good reason why a father shouldn't cover a good portion of the nighttime parenting, half if possible. Apart from breastfeeding, a father can feed, walk, or settle a baby just as well as a mother can.

Unfortunately, some men try to make the case that they have to function at work, so they should be let off the hook at night. But you also have to function during the day. If you work for pay, your job performance matters, too, and even if you don't, studies show that your hours spent in child-rearing and homemaking are probably more stressful than his are. Besides, the stakes in any day of parenting—the mind and heart of a vulnerable child—are usually more significant than whatever is on the table at work. Twenty years from now, those projects and career moves will be long forgotten, but happy and productive people will then be walking the earth thanks to all the caring—and well-rested!—attention their parents were able to give them. So, if anything, you need *more* sleep than your partner does.

If he doesn't understand this on his own, your best chance of getting your message across lies in feeling clear in your heart that he should pull his weight at night, and making your case in a serious and determined way. If he still won't do his share, that suggests larger problems, which are discussed in chapters 6 and 7.

Sleep when the baby does. If you are staying home during the day, do your best to sleep when the baby does. You may need someone to watch any older children; try to arrange this if possible. It may also mean cutting back on housework, but your sleep is more important than a tidy home!

Consider shifting the father's sleep schedule. Sometimes the solutions are a lot easier than we think; they just take a little flexibility and a willingness to try something new. For example, when their children were little, Rick started going to bed early with Jan and the kids, and then got up at 4 or 5 a.m. to work on his PhD dissertation. This helped Jan get to sleep soon enough to survive nighttime parenting, and it gave her and Rick time in bed with each other.

Ask your partner to take the baby in the early morning. By doing this, you could get more sleep while Dad can spend more time with his child. After an hour or two, the baby might be ready for a nap with Mommy, letting you have a really long stretch of dozing or sleep. Again, this will take some arranging, but it's often a pretty simple change.

Tailor sleeping arrangements to the unique needs of your family. It's easy to feel pressured to take the advice of experts or other parents on sleeping arrangements, but what's important is to choose a method that feels right to you and your partner. Each of the main approaches—baby in the parents' bedroom (co-sleeping) or down the hall—has its pluses and minuses. Co-sleeping worked for Jan and Rick's family for years, yet Ricki found that both she and her daughter got more rest once Leah was sleeping sweetly in her own room.

The bottom line is that a particular arrangement may work for one child but not her brother, or for a parent at one time but not another. It's also important to consider the context in which sleeping occurs: other children, number of bedrooms, jobs, parental illness, and so on. You may be able to adjust one of those external factors, such as work hours, in order to have the sleeping option you'd like most, or you may realize that you have to live with a less preferred sleeping arrangement for the sake of the greater good of yourself and your family. Your best guide is your own instinct and intuition, and don't let anyone—whether a know-it-all relative or a well-intentioned professional—talk you out of your deepest sense of what you, your child, and your family need. Nor is there any call to feel guilty: You will have thoroughly considered your options and made the best possible choice you could.

When the Baby Is Sleeping but You're Not

> *I often feel a spiritual communion with all the other mothers who are feeding their babies in the still of the night. Having a baby makes me feel a general closeness with humanity.*
>
> Simone Bloom

Usually by the end of a child's first or second year, she's sleeping through the night (Yes! Yes! Yes!). But many mothers still have a hard time falling asleep in the first place, or toss and turn in the middle of the night, or wake up early and are unable to get back to sleep. Thankfully, there are plenty of effective steps you can take to sleep well again.

Watch what you eat. Some moms feed the kids first but then eat a big meal later in the evening that can make their stomachs restless midway through the night; see if you can finish eating at least three hours before going to bed. You might also try reducing or eliminating caffeine, especially in the latter half of the day. Alcohol may initially relax you, but it can wake you later on. Even chocolate isn't so good right before bed, since it contains caffeine-like substances that are stimulating. Finally, don't take stimulating supplements, such as B-vitamins or ginseng, in the evening.

Lower your stress. Sleep disturbance is one sign that a person is overly stressed. For example, cortisol hormone normally rises in the morning to prepare you for the activities of the day, but with too much stress, this hormone will kick into gear extra early, waking you at 3 or 4 a.m. The primary solution is to do whatever is necessary to lower stress overall, using the tools in chapters 2 and 3. Additionally, it may be possible to reduce cortisol directly with supplements described in the next chapter. Other than a life or death emergency, *nothing* is more important for a mother than getting enough sleep.

Get exercise. Exercising in the morning or right after work can bring good sleep at night. But be careful about exercising in the later parts of the evening since that can stimulate your body and make it harder to fall asleep.

Relax your body. One mother offered this suggestion: *I find that taking a nice warm bath at night with our child really relaxes us both. It's a signal to our bodies and minds that it's time for bed.* Once you're in bed, try one or more of the relaxation techniques in chapter 2.

Use psychological techniques. Many of these methods can help you sleep better:

- Do mentally restful activities during the hour or so before bedtime, such as reading casually, listening to something soothing, or taking a bath.
- Avoid screen time an hour before bed, since late-night scrolling can keep your brain keyed up.
- Try to avoid arguments just before bed. You and your partner could agree that it's all right to table a discussion until the next day.
- Sit in a sleeping child's bedroom for a while, watching him or her breathe, and let your thoughts relax and wander.
- Meditate before bed, even for just a few minutes.
- Keep a pad and pen by your bedside to write down any thoughts or reminders for the next day, so you can get them out of your head.
- If nagging worries push forward in your mind when you settle down to sleep, like imps slipping past weary guards, make an agreement with yourself that you will think about them the next day. Also, try the techniques for dealing with anxiety discussed in the previous chapter.
- Extend compassion toward yourself. This alone can open the velvet trapdoor to sleep. You might reflect on how hard you work and how good it would feel to bring kindness to yourself, just as you do with your children.
- One of the hardest times to fall asleep is when you are mad at the person lying next to you. After focusing on compassion for yourself, you could try extending it to him. Compassion doesn't mean that you agree with him or renounce your rights, but that you are aware of his stresses and challenges, and let

yourself feel a basic kindness toward him. If you like, you could express your compassion in simple statements in your mind, such as "May Daniel be at peace" or "May Daniel and I be at peace with each other."

- Try imagining that you are breathing your love for your child in and out through your heart, or love for the child that still exists within yourself.

Supplements. Before we say another word here, we need to make an important point: *Women who are pregnant (or might become pregnant in the next few months), are breastfeeding, or have a liver disease should not take any hormones, herbs, or amino acids without being in the care of a licensed health professional experienced in their use.* And even if you're not pregnant or nursing, we always encourage you to double-check our suggestions with experienced professionals. This is the context for everything we say about supplements in this book.

Magnesium is needed for quality sleep, and it is often low in mothers. Its daily value (DV)* is 320 mg per day (360 mg if you are pregnant). As you'll see later on, we suggest that mothers consider taking somewhat higher levels of many nutrients than the DVs; we call these the mother's suggested daily value (MSDV). The MSDV for magnesium is 500 mg. Since many busy people find it difficult to get even the DV of 320 mg in their diet, you could take a supplement in the form of magnesium glycinate, lysinate, aspartate, or citrate. (Magnesium citrate tends to have a laxative effect; the other forms do not.)

Calcium is another mineral that can help you sleep better, and its DV is 1,000 mg. Calcium and magnesium are often combined in a single supplement.

---

* The minimum amount a person should consume each day.

Melatonin is a hormone secreted by the pineal gland that signals the body to sleep, and taking some just before bed could help you get a good night's rest. It can be taken sublingually (beneath the tongue) for a quick effect if it's hard to fall asleep in the first place, or swallowed in time-release form if you are troubled by nighttime waking. Some people find that taking a little sublingual melatonin immediately if they wake up in the middle of the night puts them back to sleep. If you try melatonin, find the minimum amount that works for you. Dosages as low as 0.3 to 0.5 mg can be sedating; do not exceed 3 mg, and check with your doctor if you are currently using cortisone.

Valerian and passionflower are herbs that can help bring or deepen sleep, and they are often mixed together in tinctures available in natural food stores. Herbalists also use skullcap, oat straw, and lavender. Also, the Chinese formula suan zao ren tang might aid your sleep; you can get it from an acupuncturist or some health food stores.

Serotonin is a neurochemical that helps you sleep, and the body builds it from tryptophan, an amino acid. One way to increase serotonin for sleep is to take 500 to 1,000 mg of tryptophan before bed. It must be taken on an empty stomach—so no eating for 2 to 3 hours before going to sleep. If you have a hard time going back to sleep when you wake up in the middle of the night, you could take 500 mg of tryptophan at that time.

Acupuncture. This technique consists of placing super-thin needles into specific points on a person's body, based on the Chinese theory of energy meridians. It has been used for several thousand years, and modern research has shown it to be helpful with many ailments, including pain, stroke, depression, and disturbed sleep. Since the emphasis in Chinese medicine is on healing ailments by balancing the whole body, you may find that acupuncture for insomnia provides other benefits as well.

Ask Your Doctor

If these interventions don't help, you should speak with your doctor. Online symptom checkers and AI tools can make mistakes and are no substitute for being seen by a licensed physical health practitioner.

Perhaps an illness is disturbing your sleep, such as a hormonal disturbance, diabetes, or clinical depression. For example, a patient of Ricki's, Dutonne, came for her first visit since her baby was born, looking extremely pale, worn out, and depressed. She said: *I'm just not sleeping. My head seems to bounce off the pillow when I lie down, my mind's in a whir, and there's a pounding in my ears like a drum beating.* As it turned out, the mild anemia (shortage of iron) she had during pregnancy had worsened when she bled heavily after the birth. So busy with her baby and getting everything organized, Dutonne grabbed snacks on the run and didn't get much iron in her diet. But now her heart had to race—keeping her awake at night—because her blood was less able to carry oxygen. By eating iron-rich foods and taking iron supplements, Dutonne soon felt—and was sleeping—much better.

Lack of sleep can become a vicious cycle, and with your doctor you may want to discuss sleeping pills or certain antidepressants that aid sleep. But please ask about their potential side effects. In particular, if you are nursing or could be pregnant, you should not take *any* medication, including sleeping pills, without your physician's knowledge.

A Mother's Lullaby

Ask your partner to do their share at night.

If you can, sleep when the baby does during the day.

Try sleeping arrangements that work for you.

Exercise routinely.

Have the last hour before sleeping be peaceful.
Thoroughly relax your body in bed.
Reschedule any worries to the morning.
Get enough calcium and magnesium.
Consider melatonin, herbs, other supplements, and acupuncture.
Consult your physician if you continue to have trouble with sleep.

EATING RIGHT

A baby is God's opinion that the world should go on.
Carl Sandburg

The single most effective way to replenish your body is through good nutrition. Unfortunately, most of us have a diet that is very different from the one we are adapted to through millions of years of biological evolution, which was mostly meats, vegetables, fruits, and nuts. People began eating dairy products and whole grains just ten thousand years ago—a blip on the evolutionary time scale. And it's only the last few generations that have seen the widespread use of refined grains, sugars, and oils, as well as pesticides, packaged foods, and artificial ingredients. Meanwhile, fast-food restaurants have spread widely, emphasizing the same sorts of foods: quick, processed, and super-sized with fat, sugar, and other carbohydrates, plus manufactured chemicals.

Although in the short run some people seem able to get away with this diet without too many bad consequences, the statistics on the rising incidence of type 2 diabetes, obesity, and other lifestyle-related illnesses are cautionary for anyone. This is true in general—and it's extra true for a mother, since *bearing, breastfeeding, and rearing a child are physiologically demanding activities like no others.* Doing them while staying healthy requires that you honor the fundamental biology of your body and nourish it in ways that may have been less crucial before you had children. Which means eating a lot more like your great-great-Paleolithic-grandmother than having a bagel and coffee for breakfast, peanut butter and jelly sandwich at lunch, and something microwaved for dinner. It is not always easy, but mothers who have started eating better tell us that they soon experience more energy, a lift in mood, improvement in health conditions such as dry skin or PMS, and an overall sense of greater health. It's fundamentally simple: You improve your body's balance sheet by eating more healthy foods and fewer worthless or toxic ones. At every meal, trillions of molecules at a time, you'll be literally rebuilding the tissues of your body.

In the next few pages you'll find our daily "recipe," designed specifically with a mother's nutritional needs in mind. It's made up of only seven ingredients, and you need each one of them—just like the flour, salt, water, and baking powder that are all needed to make biscuits. In sum, every day you should try to eat:

1. Approximately 60 grams/day of protein, or 80 grams/day if you're nursing
2. Five to seven servings of fresh vegetables, and one to two of fresh fruits
3. Monounsaturated oils and essential fatty acids instead of refined or hydrogenated oils, or trans-fatty acids
4. Two to five servings of unrefined, varied whole grains
5. Organic foods whenever possible
6. High-potency nutritional supplements
7. Zero or very little refined sugar

There are basically two ways to shift your diet in a healthier direction: make sweeping changes all at once or work your way into it. Whichever path you take, we urge you to stay on it until you end up with truly mother-nurturing nutrition. If you slip now and then, as almost everyone does, just get back on the path at your next meal. Optimizing nutrition often takes several tries, but each time you do it, something improves. Even small changes in the right direction add up as the months go by.

Since healthy nutrition usually involves trying new things and giving up some goodies (glazed doughnuts, etc.), a person needs to understand the reasons she's doing it, which is why we explain the health benefits of each ingredient in our recipe. You could also stay motivated by paying special attention to how eating wholesome foods helps you take good care of yourself, or even makes you feel part of a great circle, offering the sustenance of maternal care and taking in the nourishment of the earth's great bounty. Eating in a healthy way provides a good model for children, too, and helps their mother stay good-humored and patient with them, even when the oatmeal starts flying.

Ingredient #1: Approximately 60 grams/day of protein, or 80 grams/day if you're nursing; protein with every meal, especially breakfast

Why

Protein provides fundamental building blocks for your body and also helps stabilize blood sugar and prevent insulin insensitivity. Our recommendations are based on those of the National Academy of Medicine. Online, you can easily find out how much protein is in the foods you eat, and get an exact calculation of the amount of protein you need, in proportion to your weight.

How

- Eat 3–4 ounces—about the size of a deck of cards—of a good source of protein at every meal.
- In particular, *eat protein at breakfast*, and you could have less of a midday crash and irritability in the afternoon. Try two

or three eggs, a large handful of almonds, or a vegetarian or meat-based sausage.

- When you want something sweet, have some protein instead, like a hard-boiled egg, hummus on crackers, or a couple tablespoons of almond butter with an apple.
- You can get protein conveniently from these foods:
  - **Non-animal-based protein.** Many people are concerned about the ethical issues of eating animal-based products. If you're a vegetarian, as each of us has been at different times, you probably know about using food combinations (such as rice and beans) for maximum protein. Since meat is the only significant source of iron and vitamin B12 available in the human diet, a vegetarian should usually take these as part of a daily supplement.
  - If you are vegan and do not consume any animal products, you must find other ways to get adequate amounts of protein in your diet. In addition to the other vegetarian suggestions here, you can add edamame, hemp seeds, green peas, miso paste, lentils, a variety of beans (kidney, black, and pinto), or nutritional yeast to your diet. Ancient grains such as amaranth, quinoa, and teff are high in protein and do not contain gluten. Amaranth and quinoa can be used in place of rice or in soups or stews. Teff can be eaten as a porridge with berries and seeds or added as a salad topping for extra crunch. For breakfast, choosing oats or sprouted-grain bread over traditional wheat bread will add to your daily protein intake as well.
  - **Nuts.** Almonds are particularly high in protein. You could get a good trail mix or make your own; just combine your favorite nuts with some unsulfured dried fruit (kids often like to help!). Nut butters are also delicious; try almond

or sesame butter instead of peanut butter if you are allergic or sensitive to peanuts. A thick layer of almond butter on a rice cake topped with apple slices is a delicious and healthy breakfast. You can also substitute almond flour for regular flour.

— **Soy.** Soybeans and related products like tofu are a good source of protein. You can add soybeans to stews or soups, or toss tofu or tempeh chunks into a stir-fry or casserole. Soy milk comes in many flavors, and you may be surprised to find that your children really like it.

— **Hummus.** This delicious spread is made from chickpeas (garbanzo beans) and sesame seeds. You can buy it in most supermarkets or make your own, lower-fat version.

— **Protein shakes.** Just put some protein powder in a blender with your favorite liquid and perhaps some fresh fruit, and voilà! You've got an instant high-protein meal. If you are going to have smoothies regularly, try different types of protein powder (such as brown rice, hemp, pea, whey, or soy) to get a good variety. Spirulina, chia seeds, nut butters, or nut milks can all be added to your smoothies to give them a protein boost.

— **Eggs.** Eggs contain very balanced proteins. You may have avoided them because of concerns about cholesterol, but studies have found that eggs do not increase the risk of heart disease, and in fact they may raise the level of HDL ("good") cholesterol. Try to get them from free-range hens on a healthy diet. If you're in a hurry, you can hard-boil eggs in advance and eat one or two at breakfast.

— **Dairy products.** Milk, cheese, and yogurt are good sources of protein but are best consumed in moderation because many people react poorly to dairy products, and keeping the gastrointestinal tract in good shape is a top priority for a mother. If you have excessive mucus, sinus infections, disturbed digestion, or dark circles under your eyes, try experimenting with eating no dairy products for a couple of weeks and see how you feel. If you have trouble with cow-based products, then cheese etc. from goats or sheep might be fine for you. If you're wondering about calcium, you can get a fair amount of it from cauliflower, broccoli, peas, and beans. But unless you're eating many cups of these vegetables every day (or several servings of sardines or salmon, which also contain lots of calcium), you'll want to make sure to take a calcium supplement if you don't eat any dairy foods.

— **Fish.** In addition to protein, salmon contains high levels of the essential fatty acids (EFAs) every mother needs (we'll discuss EFAs in depth later on). Besides eating it fresh, you can find salmon canned or as jerky in many health food stores. Try to minimize fish at the top of the ocean food chain—like tuna, shark, or swordfish—because mercury and other toxins increase as you move up the chain.

— **Lean meat.** If you eat meat, try to get lean cuts to decrease saturated fats and the toxins that concentrate in fat. For convenience, many health food stores sell different kinds of tasty "jerkies" made from beef or turkey, and without any nitrites.

Ingredient #2: 5–7 servings of fresh vegetables and 1–2 of fresh fruits

WHY

Vegetables are just about the only thing that all nutritionists agree on, and they all say that you should eat a lot! Vegetables are rich in vitamins and minerals, and they contain phytonutrients such as carotenes and bioflavonoids, as well as phytoestrogens, hormone-like substances that seem to help balance the endocrine system. The US Department of Agriculture recommends that everyone have five servings a day (a serving is ½ cup for most vegetables, or 1 cup for leafy greens). But since you have special needs as a mother, we recommend two additional servings, for a total of seven per day. So when you tell your kids to eat their veggies, that means you too!

We recommend fresh vegetables because they have more nutrients than ones that are canned, dried, or frozen. If you can't get them fresh, frozen is your next best option—and freeze-dried vegetables make great snacks. Fresh fruits are also nourishing, filled with vitamins, phytonutrients, and fiber. But most are also very sweet, so they are best eaten in moderation (see the discussion of sugar later on).

How

- Eat a variety of high-quality vegetables, especially roots (carrots, beets), crucifers (broccoli, cauliflower), dark greens (kale, collard, spinach), and sea veggies (kelp, kombu, nori).
- Eat raw vegetables when you can (washed well). Sliced carrots, broccoli florets, and cauliflower nuggets are delicious and surprisingly sweet.
- Make several days' worth of vegetable snacks at a time, stored in plastic bags in the refrigerator. If you combine them with whole-grain rolls or pretzels, almonds, chunks of cheese, or jerkies, you can avoid prepackaged snack packs. This is one way that Ricki survived her residency and long days at the hospital delivering babies.
- Enrich salads by adding grated carrots, beets, or dark leafy greens. It's also easy to make a little extra salad for dinner, then refrigerate it in a plastic bag or container without dressing to have with lunch the next day.

- Try a "green drink" from your health food store for a serious blast of nutrients. (Pregnant or nursing moms should check with a health practitioner if it contains herbs, or find a green drink without herbs and go lightly.) Or with a sturdy blender, you can have a vitalizing elixir in just a few minutes. If it's strong enough to make your hair stand on end and your toes curl—the feeling we get from some veggie tonics—then you know it's good for you! And you can dilute it if you like.
- Cooking can make vegetables easier to digest, but that takes some time, so we like to keep it simple. Try steaming 4 cups of chopped veggies in the morning and eat them throughout the day. A baked sweet potato with a couple of eggs makes an excellent breakfast; if your oven has a delayed timer, you could pop it in the night before and wake up to a delicious aroma. Substituting sweet potatoes or yams for regular potatoes provides variety, plus additional carotenoids and other nutrients.
- We like to make a big pot of hearty vegetable soup on the weekend that could last most of the week, perhaps adding some kale or other dark, leafy greens that may taste too strong when they're raw but are milder in soup. If you toss in some protein, you've got a wonderfully nutritious meal (several, in fact!) in a pot. See the box for a recipe for our own Happy, Healthy Mom Stew.
- The best way to eat fruit is when it is fresh and whole, rather than canned, frozen, or in juice.
- Cooked fruits—such as baked apples with a little maple syrup on them, or berries with a cobbler topping—make a wholesome, delicious dessert.
- Fresh fruits and vegetables are foods that are still alive. Every time you eat or cook them, you can take a moment to sense

that the living energy within them is entering your body, giving you a feeling of peace and connection with the gifts of the earth, and a serving of stress relief with every meal.

Happy, Healthy Mom Stew: Cook Once a Week and Eat Well Every Night

The plan is to make a giant stew—10–12 quarts—that will last for a week. It will include tons of vegetables, some protein, and other goodies. When it's all cooked, put half of it in several containers in the freezer. Each stew is unique, depending on the particular ingredients on hand when it's made, but they all follow this basic framework.

1. In a big soup pot, sauté in olive oil:
   a couple of large onions, chopped
   and/or some peeled garlic cloves
   and/or some peeled and diced fresh ginger
   and/or some seasonings you like, such as fresh or dried basil, oregano, or rosemary, or ground cumin.
2. Add and sauté 2–6 pounds of protein in bite-size pieces:
   tofu (marinated and/or baked, if you like)
   or boneless, skinless chicken
   or lean beef.
3. When the protein is browned, add liquid up to about two-thirds of the pot:
   broth (vegetable, chicken, or beef)
   and/or tomato sauce
   and/or dry red or white wine (cooking evaporates the alcohol).

4. If you've used stewing beef, let it simmer for a couple of hours, until the meat is tender.
5. Starting with the ones that take longer to cook, add 8 or more cups of chopped vegetables, such as carrots, beets, squash, broccoli, green beans, peas (fresh or organic frozen), potatoes, whatever! Include several cups of chopped dark leafy greens, like kale or spinach, and try adding some dried seaweed like kombu, arame, or nori for extra mineral nourishment.
6. You can add grains (rice, barley, quinoa, pasta) or beans to the stew, or serve it over or alongside these foods. If you want to put them in, precook them or have enough extra liquid to allow for absorption. Check online for the beans you want to use since many must be precooked or presoaked; or you can use organic canned beans.
7. Many kids like broth, and a lot of nutrients from the protein and vegetables will have slipped invisibly into that liquid. If they like the broth but won't eat any vegetables, try pureeing some of the cooked vegetables in a blender and then adding them back to the soup. Sneaky . . . !

Ingredient #3: Unrefined oils and essential fatty acids instead of refined or hydrogenated oils or trans-fatty acids

Why

The process of refining oils uses toxic chemicals to strip away good nutrients while often leaving potentially harmful, altered oils behind. When oils are hydrogenated—as they are to make margarine—or kept at high temperatures for long periods of time (as in deep-fat frying), trans-fatty acids are formed, and these "bad fats" have been implicated in cardiovascular disease and other health conditions.

Essential fatty acids (EFAs) are "good fats" needed for the membranes of your cells and a healthy heart. These oils are called *essential* because they cannot be synthesized by the body and must be consumed through foods or supplements. Unfortunately, they are often deficient in mothers since they are drawn on heavily to grow a baby during pregnancy and breast milk is loaded with them, and many women don't have anywhere near enough to start with. In her practice, Jan has found that mothers typically have a stronger response to supplementing omega-3 oils than to adding any other nutrient, probably because these oils are both so important and so often deficient in mothers.

How

- Monounsaturated oils are optimal for everyday use. Virgin olive oil is good for everyday unheated or low-temperature cooking. Avocado oil is a better alternative for high-temperature frying because it has a higher smoke point.
- Avoid trans-fatty acids. These are found in deep-fried foods as well as in the hydrogenated or partially hydrogenated fats used in margarine, and in some baked or packaged foods. At home, use judicious amounts of butter or olive oil instead of margarine. At the store, check the labels, and try not to get products with these oils.
- Balance the two main types of essential fatty acids, omega-3 and omega-6. Most people are deficient in omega-3 oils yet have an oversupply of omega-6s. To put this point in perspective, throughout most of human history, people ate these oils in a ratio of approximately 1:1. But today, the average is about *16:1* omega-6s to omega-3s! That's completely out of whack

with the way our bodies are built, and one of the results is a greater tendency toward inflammation—to which mothers are already vulnerable.

The simple solution is to decrease the omega-6 oils in your diet and increase the omega-3s. The easiest way to eat less omega-6s is to stop using the oils that contain them: safflower, sunflower, soybean, and sesame oils. And then you can get more omega-3 oils in these ways:

— Eat omega-3-rich fish (salmon, mackerel, trout, or sardines). Do not overcook, or the oils will be compromised.
— Take about 1,000 mg of a fish oil supplement* that has been checked for purity, since fish (especially those at the top of the food chain) may have contaminants.
— As a vegetarian alternative to fish-based sources of EFAs, you can meet your daily needs with about 1 tablespoon of flaxseed oil, which you can add to blended or juiced drinks, or simply take in a quick gulp; flaxseed oil is also available in capsules at health food stores. You could use flaxseed oil in salad dressings and other nonfrying oil uses (essential fatty acids are degraded or destroyed at the temperatures oils reach during frying), and you might like to mix it with olive oil for flavor. Since many of us lack some of the enzymes or cofactors needed to convert flax oil into the long-chain fatty acids the body needs, which are already present in fish, make sure you're taking a good multivitamin/mineral supplement as well, for the cofactors it contains.

---

* The blood-thinning effect of fish oils may be beneficial for the cardiovascular system, much like an aspirin a day. But if you are on a blood-thinning medication or have a bleeding disorder, please consult with your doctor before supplementing with EFAs.

— Consider a gamma-linolenic acid (GLA) supplement if you have symptoms that suggest a deficiency in this nutrient, such as premenstrual tension, eczema, or arthritis. Even though GLA is an omega-6 oil, it's an exception to the general rule of minimizing omega-6 oils. The reason is that a person—especially if she's at all depleted—may lack the enzymes or nutrients needed to build GLA within the body. You can find GLA in supplements of primrose, borage, or black currant oil. Usually borage oil is the most economical while being equally effective. Some women choose to begin with the labeled dose and consider a modest increase (up to 50 percent more) to see if it helps.

Ingredient #4: 2–5 servings of unrefined, varied whole grains

Why

Refining grains takes away the fiber and nutrients (B-vitamins, etc.) present in the outer hull, but you need these to keep your GI tract running smoothly and to meet the increased stresses and energy demands that come with having children. Refined grains (e.g., white flour, pasta, white rice) also convert quickly to sugars in the body, further straining an insulin system that is already challenged by stress.

Grains definitely have a place in well-balanced nutrition. But they don't need to dominate your plate and crowd out other kinds of carbohydrates and nutrients. Plus, certain chemicals within grains called phytates can interfere with the absorption of minerals. It's also important to eat a variety of grains besides wheat, because other grains (sometimes as sources of flour)—such as rice, barley, millet, quinoa, corn, or soy—provide other nutrients, as well as the complementary amino acids needed for maximum protein. Varying your grains also lowers the chance of digestive problems or inflammation, since wheat is among the foods that people are most often allergic or sensitive to.

How

- Increase your carbohydrate intake from other sources, such as yams, vegetables, fruits, nuts, etc.
- Try to get the majority of your grains intact, not ground up in flours that convert rapidly to sugars during digestion. These could be fresh oatmeal for breakfast, a side dish of millet or quinoa at lunch, or a casserole with brown rice at dinner.
- If you have an allergy or sensitivity to wheat, try rice, millet, almond, buckwheat, sorghum, amaranth, teff, arrowroot, chickpea, coconut, tapioca, cassava, tigernut, quinoa, or corn flour products as alternatives.
- Most of us do alright with having the occasional treat made from white flour, but try not to bring home white flour products in bulk (e.g., packaged noodle or rice foods, pasta, white bread, frozen pizza, cake).
- Replace white flour with good-tasting whole wheat pastry, rice, or almond flours.
- Try pasta made from brown rice or chickpeas. There are some excellent brands that are delicious and could leave you feeling lighter than if you'd eaten wheat.

Ingredient #5: Organic foods whenever possible

Why

Organic foods have fewer toxic molecules because they contain no pesticides or artificial fertilizers. The "safety" of those chemicals has usually been established through short-term studies using single substances, often on laboratory animals. The actual experiment, though, is being carried out on human beings who consume many chemicals in combination for a lifetime. Anyone who is developing rapidly or is vulnerable—such as a child or a pregnant, stressed, or depleted mother—is particularly likely to be affected by the mounting accumulation of potentially toxic molecules.

Organic foods also tend to contain more nutritious molecules—especially minerals—because they typically come from richer soil. And besides being a two-part prescription for a mother's health—fewer bad molecules and more good ones—organic foods often taste better.

How

- Avoid foods with artificial ingredients such as preservatives, colors, or flavor enhancers. This will have the additional benefit of steering you away from the packaged foods that are loaded with white flour, hydrogenated oils, and salt.
- These days, you can get almost any food product you want from organic sources, including pasta, soup, macaroni and cheese, milk, ketchup, eggs, and even wine. Besides finding them in natural food stores, they are increasingly available in regular supermarkets. Farmers' markets are another source, plus they can be an easier place to shop with young children. Food co-ops may have organic foods, and they're a good way to meet other parents.
- Nobody should drive herself crazy to eat strictly organic foods, since a single episode—whether it's lunch at McDonald's or a salad of organic greens—doesn't make a big difference either way. It's the accumulation over time that counts.
- Organic foods are definitely more expensive, and these additional costs need to be weighed against their potential long-term benefits for you and your family. To help make your choices, check out ewg.org for their research-based guide to the foods with especially high pesticide residues (e.g., strawberries).

There's no way around it: Preparing wholesome meals from fresh ingredients takes longer than popping a frozen meal into the oven or opening a can of stew. If you're reluctant to spend more time in the kitchen, the reasons may be nothing more than feeling too busy, or cooking bores you. But sometimes a woman has mixed feelings about walking too closely in the footsteps of her own mother, or taking on some of the trappings of a traditional housewife. If that has a ring of truth for you, please take a look at the story in the box.

Kitchen Slave or Domestic Goddess?

Molly came to her appointment complaining of feeling run-down, and Ricki asked her what she was eating these days. Molly shrugged and said, *We're loaded with baby foods, crackers, pretzels, and cereals. Or we get burgers or pizza for takeout. But the produce aisle and I are strangers. I just don't want to cook.* Then she added pensively, *My mom seemed to be in the kitchen all the time when I was a kid. She never worked outside the home, like a lot of women then, and I thought she was trapped in the kitchen. When I got older, I think I looked down on her for that.* She shook her head in an embarrassed way. *I love her, but I never wanted to be stuck in the kitchen like her, with her kind of life, mostly washing and cleaning and cooking for her family. I'm leery of the classic role of being a housewife, becoming a kitchen slave, dependent on some guy. It's hard to make myself do any kind of meal planning or major grocery shopping. I'm afraid I'll get trapped too.*

Ricki nodded and agreed with Molly that it can be hard to shift gears from home to a job and then back again, and challenging to step into long-overdue opportunities for women while not throwing out the domestic arts with the dishwater.

But there's no reason a woman today can't explore both worlds. Ricki told Molly about a time when she baked gingerbread cookies for a meeting of women doctors at her house. One of them smelled the great aroma and exclaimed, *Here you're being a domestic goddess while also hosting this meeting. I've never experienced these together: comfortable cooking and the medical profession!* It became a topic of conversation in their meeting: how these busy women could let themselves be as nourished at home as at work, and as skillful in one sphere as they were in the other.

Molly went home, dusted off a cookbook, and began trying one new recipe a week. She started shopping on the edges of the supermarket and stayed out of the middle where the tempting convenience foods were concentrated. She watched a couple of cooking shows with her husband, and they enjoyed making dinner together in the happy, relaxed atmosphere they had in their kitchen.

Ingredient #6: High-potency nutritional supplements

WHY

Food has benefits that supplements don't, and supplements have benefits that foods don't. Certainly, the best sources of nutrients are usually fresh, whole, organic foods. But in real life, not some textbook, most people rely on quick snacks, meals on the run, and processed foods that lack even the DVs of all the nutrients they need. Additionally, many women already have significant nutritional deficits when they start their first pregnancy.

Plus, we think you need more than the DVs anyway! Growing and nursing a baby, as well as the hard work and stress of raising a family, drain nutrients from a woman's body. But it's hard to match that increased outflow with an inflow of nutrients since gastrointestinal disturbances (common among mothers) impair their absorption. Building up reserves in your body is an insurance policy against future times of high stress or poor nutrition.

Further, the DVs are the *minimum* necessary to prevent diseases of nutritional deficiency, not necessarily what promotes long-term health and well-being. For example, the amount of vitamin C that prevents scurvy is less than that which brings the greatest cardiovascular health across a lifetime. A growing body of research has substantiated the benefits of above-DV levels of various nutrients for gastrointestinal dysfunction, depression, hormonal disturbances, and autoimmune diseases—for which women have an increased risk after children. (Of course, supplements are no substitute for a balanced diet or medical care.)

How

- Unless your doctor has instructed you otherwise due to a specific medical condition, we suggest that you take multivitamin/mineral supplements whose dosages meet the criteria of our mother's suggested daily values (MSDVs) listed in Appendix C. (If you are pregnant or breastfeeding, or have delivered or weaned a child in the past year, Appendix C also lists the increased amounts of certain nutrients you need.) We also list the intensive daily doses (IDDs) that may help with specific health conditions. Do not exceed the IDDs unless you have been specifically instructed to do so by a licensed health practitioner. In particular, to avoid harmful effects on a developing fetus, do not take more than 5,000 IU of vitamin A if you are pregnant, planning to get pregnant in the next couple of months, or having sex without contraception.

Your prenatal vitamin/mineral supplements may be all you need, but check the labels; many have levels of important nutrients that are too low. Health food stores usually carry several brands of high-quality multis that meet most or all of our MSDVs. Whether you're taking an everyday multi or a more exotic nutrient, always be sure to get supplements with guaranteed purity and potency from reputable companies.

- Use a supplement whose minerals are chelated, which aids absorption. This is indicated when the name of the mineral is followed by a word ending in *-ate*, such as citrate, aspartate, malate, gluconate, or picolate. (Chelated minerals are also usually a sign of a quality product; magnesium ox*ide*, for instance, is cheap to manufacture, but it's not absorbed as well.) If you can't get iron in a chelated form, look for ferrous—not ferric—sulfate, fumarate, or gluconate.
- You will probably need to add calcium and magnesium to even the best multi in order to get the amounts of these minerals that you need.
- You may also want to take an additional B-complex supplement. All the B-vitamins help people deal with stress. For example, B5 enables the body to make adrenal hormones. Vitamin B6 helps balance the endocrine system; this vitamin often helps with PMS, morning sickness, and depression.
- If you are breastfeeding or have weaned your child in the past year, you might consider taking 500 mg of the amino acid taurine with your breakfast. (This is the exception to our general recommendation that you take no amino acid supplements if you are breastfeeding or pregnant unless you've been otherwise instructed by a licensed health professional.) Because taurine plays an important role in infant development, some practitioners suggest that nursing can place extra demands on a

mother's taurine supply. Taurine also supports healthy mineral balance within your body's cells—particularly magnesium, which is necessary for sleep, relaxation, and vitality.

- Expect to take a handful of pills each day, since there is no way that all the micronutrients you need can fit into a single supplement smaller than a hefty marble. This takes less time than brushing your teeth, and it could be as important for your overall health in the long run.

Ingredient #7: Zero or very little refined sugar

Why

Sure, when we're blue or want some comfort or just a jump start, most of us like to have something sweet to eat. Initially, refined sugar does bring a blast of energy. But the spike in blood sugar triggers a big surge of insulin in the body's effort to get all that sugar into your cells. Then the wave of insulin does its job so well that your blood sugar levels quickly plummet. Suddenly you feel hungry, spacey, fatigued, jittery, shaky, short-tempered, or even panicky.

Clearly, these are not the desired effects of a sugar buzz! Even worse, our cells become less sensitive to insulin over time as a self-protective measure. That makes the pancreas pump out extra insulin, which makes our cells even less sensitive. It's a vicious cycle. If this process continues, at some point the pancreas just can't pump out enough insulin to get the cells to take notice, and now a person has type 2 diabetes.

The average American today eats 60–70 pounds per year of refined sugars—compared to zero pounds during most of human history. High consumption of sugar (and the elevated levels of insulin that come with it) is associated with type 2 diabetes, weight gain, bloating, fatigue, arthritis, migraines, lowered immune function, gallstones, obesity, breast cancer, and cardiovascular disease. And sugar is depleting, the last thing a mother needs, draining (or disrupting the absorption of) the B-vitamins, chromium, calcium, magnesium, and copper that she needs to manage her increased stresses. Sugar also feeds some of the microbes in the digestive tract, which can lead to impaired nutrient absorption, diarrhea, gas, or fatigue.

How

- Sugar has an addictive quality: When you have a little, you want more. So for some people, cutting out sugar altogether is the only way to go. If that's too radical, we suggest you set a personal goal of eating less than 20 grams of refined sugar a day (about 5 teaspoons). If you have any digestive problems, we think you should eat no more than 10 grams a day. Food labels will tell you how many grams of refined sugar a serving contains, and it probably doesn't much matter if it's refined or "natural" (like fructose or honey).
- An easy way to eat less sugar is to cut out soda, juice, or fancy sweetened coffee drinks. Drinking two soft drinks a day will add about 70 *pounds* of sugar to your diet each year. Instead, try flavored seltzer, carbonated water with a squeeze of lemon or lime, or delicious herbal iced teas.
- Check the labels on packaged foods like breakfast cereal, peanut butter, or spaghetti sauce, and try brands without any sugar.
- Think twice about extra sugar, like a second teaspoon in your coffee, tons of jam on toast, or an extra helping of ice cream after dinner.
- By having fewer sweets around for your kids, it will be easier to avoid them yourself.
- Avoid temptation by not having cookies, candy, ice cream, etc. at home. If you want something for your sweet tooth, purchase

a single item. And if you do keep dessert around, try to have only one kind, since we tend to eat more if there's a variety.

- If you are, like Jan, a chocolate fanatic, try high-quality unsweetened chocolate. Once you get used to it, it tastes very satisfying. You can melt it, add a couple drops of stevia and a handful of nuts, and make your own candy bar.
- Try to understand the forces that keep you hooked on sugar. For instance, Jan worked with a single mom who ate a huge, double handful of chocolate chips each day. She knew it wasn't healthy, but she said: *I know it's not good, but I work hard all day long, and this is about the only thing I do for* me. By finding better ways to nurture herself, she was able to cut down on this daily blast of sugar.
- Sugar is the ultimate comfort food, so it's really important to be nice to yourself while you reduce it. And try to think about all the wonderful things you are doing for your body by nourishing it in healthier ways.

I can resist everything except temptation.

Oscar Wilde

EXERCISING REGULARLY

Samantha, a patient of Ricki's, came to her appointment concerned about her weight, which was still more than 20 pounds heavier than it had been before having her first baby, now three years old. Ricki asked about exercise, and Samantha smiled and quoted a saying: *Oh, I do get the urge sometimes. But I just lie down until it passes!* Then she became more serious and added, *I just can't find the time. My day is busy from 6 a.m. to 11 at night.* Ricki wondered about her husband,

and Samantha explained, *Ben jogs from 6 to 6:45 every morning, then showers, bolts down his breakfast, and is out of the house by 7:30.* The gears began to turn. *You're right,* she mused, *he makes it a priority. Why don't I?*

They talked about how exercise has to be important, or it just won't happen. As a result, Samantha went home and had a long talk with Ben, and he agreed to take over childcare and dinner preparation three nights a week. Samantha began jogging on a treadmill in the bedroom while watching the evening news. Ben enjoyed becoming more than a "microwave chef," and he liked spending more time with their daughter, who stood on top of a step stool helping him with nightly lettuce tearing and salad tossing. In a year, Samantha lost 22 pounds, felt more energetic, and had a sunnier mood.

To motivate yourself, remember that exercise will improve your cardiovascular health, strengthen your immune system, and help prevent obesity and type 2 diabetes. It brings vitality, energy, and relaxation and lifts depressive feelings. Think about your reasons for taking good care of yourself, like wanting to live a long and healthy life. None of us really "finds" time for self-care and exercise. We *make* time for these crucial activities because they are essential to our well-being as well as to the health and happiness of those around us.

You probably already have an idea of what kind of exercise you'd do if you only had the time. And if not, you can get tons of information about exercise online. If you've recently had a baby, your OB/GYN can make recommendations about safe and gentle exercises to strengthen stretched-out abdominal muscles or tighten up your pelvic floor. Of course, if you have any orthopedic or anatomic problems that interfere with exercise, please consult your doctor or physical therapist for specific suggestions. The key issue is typically *how* to shoehorn exercise into a day that's already crowded with work and family. That's our focus here, as we look at ways to fit fitness into everyday life with children.

Getting Started

If you are just starting to exercise, take heart. It feels great simply to begin, to know that, yes, you are really doing something wonderful for yourself. Set realistic goals that you know you can consistently attain, and perhaps write them down so you can see them every day and stay on track with your *own* care amid attention-grabbing care of others.

A regular exercise buddy or class could help you stay motivated. If your resolve starts to sag, take a look at that picture of yourself as a child we mentioned in chapter 2. She is precious and beautiful, and seeing her sweet face can help sustain your positive self-loving energy. Once you build up momentum after a few weeks, it will feel odd *not* to exercise, and every step you take on your own behalf—whether baby-sized or big ones—will make you feel better and better.

If you haven't exercised for a few months or more, take it easy when you start up again. If your body has become at all depleted, your muscles and connective tissue could be prone to strain, since they may have low levels of the minerals that keep them supple and resilient. So before you dive into a major program, we suggest you take a few days first to do 10 to 20 minutes a day of gentle yoga or stretching. And try to do some easy stretches at the start of any workout; stiff muscles are like sleeping children: They need encouragement and a little time to wake up!

Aerobic Activities

Any good fitness program balances the development of aerobic capacity and strength. Your goal is to work up to keeping your heart beating rapidly (so that you're breathing quickly and deeply but can still carry on a conversation) for at least 20 to 30 minutes, three or four times a week. No matter how out of shape you might be, or super-busy, there's always *something* you can do to get the blood moving and a sparkle in your eyes. Here are some suggestions we've seen work for mothers.

Go for a walk or a run. You can walk by yourself, grab another mom, or chat on your phone to catch up with a friend. Bringing your child in a stroller or in a baby backpack will make it even more aerobic, plus handle your childcare. In your neighborhood or community, there may be a group of mothers who go for walks together. Jan joined one of these called Babes on Their Backs that took short hikes with little ones in baby-packs. Or if you're ready to pick up the pace, you can go for a run. You could even bring your child by using a baby jogger.

Ride a bike. Riding is great fun with a child. She can sit behind you in a kid-seat, or you can get a cruiser-trailer that hooks onto the end of your bike, and she'll look like she's riding in style like a queen in a carriage. If she's old enough to ride on her own, she can come with you, though you may need to drop her off back home midway through your workout.

Take an aerobics class or use the equipment in a gym. Many gyms now have on-site childcare, even for infants. We know mothers who joined a gym with high intentions, but it was so much hassle to get out of the house that they finally gave up—so try to work out a regular schedule with your partner that's truly feasible and not rushed.

Go for a swim. Swimming is especially good for mothers who have connective tissue problems and need low-impact exercise.

In the comfort of your home. Many women like to exercise at home using live or prerecorded online classes. Or get your own treadmill, rowing machine, etc. For example, every morning Ricki reads the newspaper while riding a stationary bike at home. Beginning when Leah was in preschool, Ricki started getting up a half hour earlier to do this—and her only regret is that she didn't start a couple of months after her baby was born!

Strength Training

Many studies have shown the benefits of strength training. Of course, go at a reasonable pace and don't strain yourself.

The obvious option is to use free weights or machines in your home or a gym. But you might also be amazed at how much of a workout you can get while tending to children, running errands, or doing housework. You might try keeping a set of weights available and doing a light arm workout while you're chatting with a friend. Carry your grocery bags by their handles, so you can either curl your biceps or stiffen your elbows and challenge your shoulders by seeing how high you can raise the bags.

Just like with aerobics, there's always *something* you can do to become stronger. Making a change is usually hard at first, especially if you're already fatigued from 3 a.m. wake-ups with a young child or long days at work. It's also a sad irony that guilt about not taking steps for yourself can make you feel so down and discouraged that it's even harder to get some exercise! But when people reflect back on their lives, it is often the positive changes they have made and sustained that they feel best about. That's the best way to let go of guilt: Try one of the road-tested suggestions above, notice how good you start to feel, and go on to take another step toward your fitness improvement goals.

KEEPING A BASIC BALANCE IN YOUR LIFE

So far, we've discussed your health mainly from the perspective of Western science and medicine. But as powerful as those approaches are, the idea of overall life balance has been much more developed within an entirely different framework, that of traditional Chinese medicine (TCM). We'll apply its basic principles to three types of moms, and then we'll tell you the Chinese herbal formula that could increase the well-being of each type.

The Traditional Chinese View of Mothers

Chinese medicine—practiced for over 5,000 years—is founded on bringing harmony to the forces inside and around a person. In your own life, these would include the interplay of systems within your body, as well as the ebb and flow of your emotions. These forces are considered to exist within the Tao, the mysterious, generative unfolding of the universe, the mother of all things:

> *The Tao is called the Great Mother:*
> *empty yet inexhaustible,*
> *it gives birth to infinite worlds.*
>
> Tao Te Ching, *by Lao Tzu (English version by Stephen Mitchell)*

TCM recommends that a mother be given great care around and after the birth of her child. Since she has poured out so much during pregnancy and childbirth, balance must be restored both by arranging for her to do as little as possible and by replenishing her through rest and nourishing foods and herbs. For at least a month, the mother and her baby should be taken care of by her relatives and friends. And after that, she should continue to be nurtured with good nutrition, love, and other kinds of support.

The core concepts of Chinese medicine are less mechanistic than the variables Western doctors study, like counts of white blood cells or transfer rates across cell membranes. Rather than seeing the body as a machine, traditional Chinese doctors view it more as a dance of subtle energies. The more harmonious the dance, the healthier the dancer.

Two fundamental forces are called *yin* and *yang*. Yin is the receptive principle, and is associated with earth, darkness, yielding, rest, passivity, cold, inwardness, pause, quiet, and decrease. Yang is the active principle, associated with sky, light, firmness, activity, initiative, heat, outwardness, speed, noise, and increase. Yin is sometimes viewed as feminine and yang as masculine, although each is present in every person regardless of gender.

The symbol of yin and yang is a circle, with one portion dark for yin and one portion light for yang. But at the center of the yin is a spot of yang, and at the center of yang is a spot of yin. This maintains the balance of yin and yang. Within each principle, the opposite one is blooming. For instance, in activity there must be a center of quiet observation, and in the darkness of the night sky there must be seeds of light.

Each principle has value: The sky is not better than the earth, and cold is not better than hot. But life becomes imbalanced when a person gets carried away by one principle and lacking in the other, and this can lead to problems. For example, if you are active, afterward you need some rest. If you give attention and love all day long, you need to receive it as well.

The balance of yin and yang that is most harmonious will vary from person to person. To find the balance that is right for you, think about these questions:

- What are the yin elements within your life? What are the yang ones?
- Does the yin principle seem to be lacking? Or does it seem excessive? How about the yang principle: lacking or excessive?
- How might it be healthy for you to build up the yin in your life? Or to limit it? The same for yang: increase or decrease it?

To put these questions in a larger context, consider the balance of yin and yang in our society. Modern civilizations are very yang, and that excess in combination with a lack of yin is an underlying cause of many stress- and lifestyle-related illnesses. It's as if we all live inside a giant furnace, with the bellows of media, smartphones, corporate culture, and all the rest fanning the flames of excessive speed, activity, and clamor. To restore balance to her life, a mother often benefits from reducing these too-powerful yang forces as best she can and fostering more yin—which mothers the mother. And on this foundation, she may also benefit from boosting certain yang elements, such as asserting herself with her partner or taking initiative to find a better job.

The Mother with Depleted Yin

Now let's apply these ideas to a mom with depleted yin (some of the details won't fit every mother whose yin forces have become depleted). Laurie had always been sensitive and a little nervous, but she felt that way more than ever since becoming a mother four years ago, now with two young children. There was a background sense of being uneasy and frazzled much of the time, and seemingly little things could really upset her. It seemed hard for her to *settle*, and deep inside there was a longing for the nurturance of others, in part because it had become so hard to soothe herself. She felt frayed at the very root of her being.

Physically, Laurie sometimes felt a bit dizzy for no apparent reason, an irritating ringing in her ears came and went, and she often had low back pain. After each pregnancy, she went through many weeks of hot flashes and night sweats. She sometimes felt oddly dry no matter how much water she drank or lotion she put on. On occasion, particularly in the afternoon, she felt a sensation of heat, especially in the palms of her hands and the soles of her feet.

In Chinese medicine, depleted yin means insufficient calming, cooling, and nurturing. The body lacks the ability to absorb stress and return to equilibrium. In a sense, yin is embodied in part by the parasympathetic nervous system, which balances the sympathetic nervous system that is triggered during stress; without that regulating influence, the body is left in a continual state of "fight or flight" overdrive.

An herbal formula for depleted yin is called zhi bai di huang wan.* Its key herb is rehmania, known to the Chinese as shu di huang. Rehmania is considered to be a richly moistening and nourishing herb—very helpful for a mother with low yin.

The Mother with Depleted Qi

In the ancient Chinese system, qi—pronounced "chee" and sometimes spelled chi—is considered to be the "vital force" or subtle energy that flows in and around all life. From this perspective, qi:

- Originates and accompanies all movement, from exercise to the gyrations of atomic particles
- Protects you, which links qi, in Western thinking, to the immune system
- Provides for harmonious transformations, such as the metabolism of food into usable nutrients
- Holds things in place; for instance, prolapse of an organ would reflect a severe deficiency of qi
- Warms; a person who often feels cold probably needs more qi

* To repeat an oft-made point, women who are pregnant or might be, or who are nursing, should not take any medication or herbs without the specific approval of the relevant, licensed health practitioner.

You get your qi from the "prenatal qi" you were born with (like the charge in a battery), and from breathing, food, and herbs (like freshly generated electricity). A person cannot replenish her prenatal qi—that particular battery cannot recharge—and in Chinese medicine, motherhood is considered to irreversibly drain a large portion of a woman's prenatal qi. It is thus vital to make sure you are receiving a healthy influx of qi and that it is flowing freely.

Letitia was an example of a mother with depleted qi. She felt tired all the time, and she hadn't gotten her energy back since she had Darrin, more than two years ago. She weaned him early, since it seemed like she couldn't produce enough breast milk. She still needed to nap when he did, even though she was sleeping eight or more hours at night. Letitia had gained 15 to 20 pounds over her prepregnancy weight, but she was too tired to do anything about it. She felt physically tired much of the time, and her body would break into a light sweat from even mild exertion.

Besides feeling weary, Letitia thought her digestive system wasn't working very well anymore. She often felt bloated after meals, and she had noticed that a number of foods no longer agreed with her. Additionally, she frequently felt chilly and vulnerable, with few reserves deep inside to meet the day, and she caught just about every cold her son brought home from preschool. She bruised easily, and she often felt dizzy for a bit when she stood up.

Simply eating nutritious foods and breathing deeply would increase Letitia's qi. Additionally, in cases of moderate to severe qi deficiency, a classic Chinese formula—called bu zhong yi qi tang—is worth considering. One of the key herbs in this formula is astragalus. In Western herbal practices, astragalus is used for its energy-boosting properties and to strengthen the immune system.

The Mother with Constrained Qi

Besides being depleted, qi can be bottled up and constrained. For example, Minda had a three-year-old son and an eight-month-old daughter. She often felt frustrated, edgy, and cranky. Her PMS was very intense, with bloating, sharp irritability, glum mood, sore breasts, and cramps. She noticed herself snapping at her husband and children when they didn't deserve it. Some days, she felt wound so tight that it seemed she could explode.

Minda's qi was not moving freely, and depression and irritability were among the results. Constrained qi is also associated with menstrual problems, including irregularities in the cycle, breast tenderness, cramping, and a sense of emotional turmoil. A mother with constrained qi may have difficulty with lactation: The milk is present, but—like the qi—it does not flow freely. She may have lumpy breasts or develop mastitis (breast infection).* Headaches are common in individuals with constrained qi.

You can unblock qi simply by shifting your body into a more comfortable position, pursuing a creative interest, or expressing something you've been holding back. Additionally, you could use the Chinese formula dan zhi xiao yao san. And if this is not available, try a more general formula called xiao yao san. Either of these formulas could be helpful for any mother under high levels of stress.

REGULAR CHECKUPS

Depletion starts at the molecular level in your body, and it can go a long way before becoming really obvious. To stay healthy, you need to

---

* If you have mastitis, please see a doctor; the formulas we mention here will not treat your condition.

catch little things before they get big. Putting off checkups until you're ill is like searching the stable for clues after the horse has run away. For instance, Margie brought her two-year-old to the pediatrician and mentioned, only in passing, that she was four months pregnant but had not yet seen her obstetrician (Ricki) because she had been unable to "organize" the appointment. Margie lost her train of thought a couple times, but she reassured the doctor that she was only tired, due to still getting up at night with her daughter. Nonetheless, he was concerned about Margie and encouraged her to see her obstetrician as soon as possible. Based on Margie's fatigue, sluggish reflexes, and swelling in her lower legs, Ricki ordered blood tests for thyroid hormones, which showed low levels. Ricki prescribed a thyroid supplement, and by eight weeks later Margie felt better, and at twelve weeks, follow-up testing showed normal thyroid function.

In another case, Carolyn came to see Jan for help with her nutrition. Flustered about arriving 20 minutes late to her first appointment, she made an offhand remark about feeling these days *like there's no insulation anymore on the wiring in my brain.* She had previously managed a high-powered career with aplomb, working as a senior editor at a major newspaper. But now, small hassles looked huge, and she usually felt both tense and exhausted. In addition to receiving a routine physical exam from her family doctor, Carolyn had seen an endocrinologist, but that assessment had found no problems with Carolyn's hormones. Jan suggested testing her amino acids, and indeed, two important ones—tyrosine and taurine—had become seriously depleted. Jan arranged for Carolyn to get a balanced amino acid formula, and she began feeling much better in just a few weeks. Looking back on what had happened, she said: *I don't think I would have let things go so far before I had Chianna. You're coping with something new every day, and you're* so *tired that you just hold on and figure it'll get better. But, you know, I think I also sort of expected to feel not-great, so when I started feeling worse and worse, I thought it was normal for moms, or at least this one. If I'd had it to do all over again, I'd seek help for my health much sooner.*

Most mothers see a physician for themselves just once a year, if at all, typically at their annual gynecologist appointment. Lab studies beyond Pap smears are not routinely done unless a problem is mentioned or something during the exam raises concerns (or if you had certain health problems during a recent pregnancy). Sadly, millions of Americans cannot afford health insurance or lack access to quality health care for other reasons. Our suggestions here are meant for those who can access health care, but even if you face obstacles, it's crucial to keep advocating for your health. Persisting on your own behalf is one of the most important ways to support your long-term well-being.

Before seeing a health care provider, it's important to reflect on how you are feeling, especially if you have changed providers since your last checkup or your child's birth. Your needs matter, and health care workers can figure out what is going on and lend a helping hand only if they know how you are doing. So here are some suggestions for getting the most out of your appointment with your gynecologist or another doctor.

Keep a personal health file. It is very helpful to keep a brief diary of symptoms, lab work, office visits, or the resolution of problems as your own home medical chart. Then, if something doesn't go away on its own, you are an excellent historian when asked to describe it. We're not suggesting that you catalog every ache, pain, or blue moment. But it's important not to downplay physical or emotional problems.

Be organized for the appointment. Bring your personal health file and a list of the questions you want to address. Take notes during the appointment (or right afterward) so you can remember key points later.

Be brave. Sharing the frailties you may be experiencing can take courage. But your doctor can't know that you, let's say, are losing urine with coughing and sneezing unless you mention it. Similarly, if you feel wiped out and run down, you need to be clear with any medical staff when they interview you that this is an important item to address with the doctor.

Tell your doctor about your history and any risk factors. For example, a family history of problems with your reproductive, hormone, gastrointestinal, or nervous systems increases your risk for depletion. Heavy and frequent menstruation may drain iron or suggest an imbalance in your hormones. Difficult pregnancies or miscarriages stress a woman's body. A postpartum depression triples the risk of another one, and it may indicate underlying vulnerabilities in the endocrine system. Past experiences of depression, anxiety, trauma, or drug or alcohol abuse can suggest a sensitivity to the stresses of motherhood.

Share how you've been feeling. Let your doctor know how you are really managing emotionally while taking care of your children, home, work, and other obligations. He or she will want to know about the stressors in your life, such as a child with health problems, or relationship conflicts. You can ask for a referral to other professionals or to agencies that might help, such as a therapist, a psychiatrist for possible medication, or a parenting educator.

Bring a list of all your medications and supplements. That way, your health care providers can be aware of any interactions or side effects.

Perhaps make a special appointment. If you need to, make a separate appointment to discuss these issues, since they deserve adequate time for reflection, not the hurried type of "roller skates" doctor visit that has become so common with managed care schedules. Most physicians will be sympathetic and helpful. But if little interest is shown, you may need to look around for another doctor, since that person will be a crucial resource for your long-term health.

Follow up if necessary. Examination and history-taking alone may give you and your doctor enough information to make a sufficient assessment of your health and well-being. Based on the findings, your providers could recommend a course of action, and if it works, then that may confirm their initial diagnosis. For example, if you feel run down and have been eating poorly, a reasonable first step is to improve your diet and get more rest; if that restores your sense of vitality, there could be no need for further investigation.

But if the minimum assessment raises nagging questions, the first round of intervention has mixed results, or you simply want a thorough review of your health, then we encourage you to pursue further testing; the next chapter summarizes how to assess the gastrointestinal, nervous, endocrine, and immune systems of your body. If you take this step, please be sure to look at Appendix D for an insider's view of how to advocate for yourself in the modern health care system, and to think clearly about the assessment results and your doctor's recommendations.

Unfortunately, some health care organizations resist assessment because it costs money, and you may have to advocate for yourself to get the tests you need. At worst, you may need to pay out of pocket for some testing. As difficult as that can be, an investment in your health usually comes back tenfold in lifetime earnings, decreased medical costs, and the intangible but precious benefit of feeling good in your own body.

Of course, the purpose of assessment is to understand what action you need to take in order to feel better. In the next chapter, we will describe how you can use the information you have gained to reverse the process of depletion in your body and restore greater balance to several of its vital systems.

CHAPTER FIVE

What to Do If You're Getting Depleted

You can usually prevent the depletion of your body's resources by experiencing generally low stress and maintaining the good wellness practices we discussed in the previous chapter. But if you find that there's just no way to have a low-stress life, or you entered motherhood with a physical vulnerability, or you—like most mothers—have already undergone a year or more of serious outpouring with little replenishment, there's a good chance that you're already getting depleted—perhaps to the point of developing what we call depleted mother syndrome (DMS). So here you'll be learning about physical interventions to reverse that process and restore:

- The nutrients that keep you healthy
- Balance to the systems of your body

This chapter is different from the others. Basically, it's a repair manual full of detailed information—with an emphasis on what is relevant to mothers—about four key systems in your body: gastrointestinal, nervous, endocrine, and immune. (A person could have a health condition in another bodily system, such as musculoskeletal or cardiovascular, but we've selected the four systems that, in our experience, are most commonly depleted by motherhood.) As with any repair manual, there's not much sense in reading about whatever is working fine—unless you have a particular interest in health, especially from a holistic perspective. And if you're feeling really good in general, you could skip ahead to the next chapter.

The checkups with your doctor described at the end of the previous chapter may already have identified specific health problems and made it clear which section(s) of this chapter you should look at. Additionally, see which, if any, of the following symptoms apply to you, and that will also indicate the section(s) of this chapter that will be most helpful for you:

- **Gastrointestinal:** Overfullness or gassiness after eating, heartburn, indigestion, stomach or abdominal pain or cramping, blood or mucus in the stool, food sensitivities, frequent vaginal yeast infections, overproduction of respiratory mucus, constipation, diarrhea, irritable bowel syndrome, fatigue
- **Nervous:** Depressed mood, chronic anxiety, feeling reactive, problems sleeping, worsened concentration and memory, tremor, chronic headaches, any sudden change in cognitive function
- **Endocrine:** Fatigue, worsened PMS, feeling chilled or hot (including hot flashes), vaginal dryness, change in sexual response, dry skin, unusual hair loss, depression or anxiety, feeling hyper, heart palpitations
- **Immune:** More frequent and longer colds, cold sores, or genital herpes; new allergies or heightened reactions to known

allergens; new or heightened autoimmune reactions; chronic inflammation (e.g., painful joints)

Our focus here is on replenishing and balancing your bodily systems rather than treating any particular ailment. If you have (or suspect you might have) an illness, you should see your doctor immediately. Additionally, we recommend that you try the interventions we describe only in the context of an ongoing professional relationship with a knowledgeable, licensed health care provider—ideally one who is familiar with integrative medicine.

Since Jan developed problems in all four systems, she'll start by telling her story, which illustrates how health conditions are often intertwined, and how to address them *in combination*. Next, we will describe the spectrum of health care methods. Then, for each system, you'll learn about:

- The system in general
- How motherhood can affect it
- Common symptoms
- Tips for assessing it
- Ways to replenish and balance it

Because the long-term health of mothers has unfortunately received little attention, our suggestions are essentially a first draft of a comprehensive protocol for reversing maternal depletion. New research may suggest some revisions. We've also chosen to be conservative, generally mentioning only those interventions that have received support in the research literature, and with which we are familiar; other practitioners may suggest different methods. And you should always listen to your own intuitive wisdom as to what is best for *you*. To your health!

JAN'S STORY: "I'M GOING TO GET BETTER!"

Before having children, I had always been a healthy, basically happy person with an even-keeled disposition. That's why it was so shocking when I became increasingly depleted, even as I was feeling joyously fulfilled by motherhood. Although I've spoken with many moms who had experiences that were similar in some ways to my own, every mother's story is different; please see what fits for you in mine.

Drains and Stresses

I was 32 when I became pregnant for the first time, but after twelve weeks, I miscarried in a night of intense labor, and I was very upset at this loss. After a few months, I got pregnant again. I enjoyed my size; having always been a little overweight, it was now OK to be so! Because my baby was in a breech and oblique position, we scheduled a C-section and it went fine, and I quickly bounced back.

I felt committed to a very nurturing style of parenting. But it sure was a lot of work! I responded to Forrest quickly if he wanted something, and I nursed him whenever he was hungry. Rick loved taking care of Forrest and was very skillful at it. But since Rick was the sole provider while also going to graduate school, he wasn't around much. And no one else seemed to be around either. Our relatives all lived far away, and our circle of friends without children gradually evaporated. I felt isolated for the first time in my life. Meanwhile, I returned to part-time work at home when Forrest was just a few months old; Rick would care for him while I did a form of deep-tissue bodywork for my clients. Taken as a whole, I was pouring out a lot and handling a fair amount of stress, with very little replenishment. But so far, my health remained good, and Rick and I felt eager to have another baby.

I became pregnant with Laurel soon after Forrest turned two, and I chose to continue breastfeeding him because I felt it was the best thing for him. But the nursing, which had always gone well, started to get physically uncomfortable, a warning sign that something was out of balance, which I ignored. I continued working—and looking after a rambunctious two-year-old—until one month before Laurel was born.

Another warning sign: My relationship with Rick began to suffer during this pregnancy, for the very first time in our long relationship. I was worn out, busy with Forrest and work, and queasy most of the time, so my marriage was at the bottom of my priorities. Rick saw how much I was dragging and worried about me. He encouraged me to take more time for myself, but I just couldn't, somehow: It seemed like such a hassle to organize, and it was hard to be away from my son. When we went to the hospital to deliver Laurel via C-section (same breech problem), I became painfully aware of the gulf that had grown between us. Rick was very sweet with me while we waited to begin the procedure, and I hadn't felt that connection to him for so long. It made me deeply sad.

Laurel was a really easy baby. Nonetheless, with a single child, you occasionally get relief, but now the two of them never seemed to sleep at the same time! Each day became a long sprint of work leading up to an exhausting night. On top of that, I was now nursing both children. My body seemed to cry "no" at the thought of breastfeeding Forrest as well as Laurel, but I felt I couldn't refuse him. I was sure he would have been devastated if he lost his nursing along with having to share his mother's love and time with his sister.

Amid all this outpouring, the stresses continued to add up during that first year after Laurel's birth. With the C-section, my body had undergone its second surgical procedure in a few years. Sleep was constantly interrupted. When Rick and I argued about raising the kids, there was an intensity that had never been present before in our fights, because the issues had never been as serious. Our quarrels would rattle me for many hours afterward.

I wasn't getting replenished, and the resources in my body were low from extensive nursing and three pregnancies in a little over three years (counting the miscarriage). I ate whatever I could on the run, and when a well-meaning friend told me she got all the nutrients she needed from her foods alone, I followed her lead and stopped taking any vitamins. As to psychological resources, I had almost no time to myself. Our marriage had also grown cooler. We kept loving each other, and there were many nice times together, but it was getting all too easy to feel very disconnected.

This one-two punch of growing demands and shrinking resources was wearing on me right where I was most vulnerable. I was 36 when Laurel was born, and my body lacked the pep and resilience it had had 10 years before—let alone 20 years before, the age when women in earlier generations typically began having children. Second, as I would later discover, my gastrointestinal tract had already been disturbed by years of taking antibiotics for teenage acne, and even more years of a hefty diet of sweets.

The Crash

Trouble had been headed my way long before I saw it, like a tidal wave starting a thousand miles offshore. Unbeknownst to me, microscopic changes in my body were accumulating, and when they finally crashed into plain view, the consequences were serious. As we approached Laurel's first birthday, I acquired a chronic, daily headache that no amount of ibuprofen could eliminate, and I began to experience ongoing pain in my shoulders and back. I routinely awoke in the middle of the night and was unable to return to sleep. My whole body started feeling reactive; small scares would get my heart pounding, and it felt like the nerve endings in my brain were frayed and raw. I became uncharacteristically forgetful, I was rarely happy, little things that had never bothered me before now sent me into tears, and it took longer to recover emotionally.

Gloomy, pessimistic circles of thought captured my attention, and I became preoccupied with the alarming and unprecedented collapse in my health: *What is happening to me?!* I am a very analytical person, and it was completely frustrating not to be able to figure out why my body was falling apart.

The Realization

Finally, the first breakthrough occurred a few months after Forrest turned three. A chiropractor examined my loose connective tissue, sagging muscles, and gaunt appearance. She asked soberly, "What do you hold your baby up with, your will?" It was a great moment. I realized that instead of being a wimp, I was doing my best within a deteriorating body. Rick and I talked a lot, and he really began to understand what was going on with me in a new way. Rather than seeing me as someone who, unaccountably, just couldn't get it together to keep the house straight while he was working hard and studying for his licensing exams, he now realized that I was struggling with a *physical* condition. And around this time I weaned Forrest, which he accepted.

A second breakthrough soon followed. I had arranged for a babysitter to watch Laurel while I went to the mall with Forrest. This was supposed to be a fun time, when I got to do three of my favorite things: be with my son, window shop, and have something sweet to eat. But I walked around the mall with absolutely no interest in shopping, and when I bought Forrest and myself some ice cream, I just stared at my cone numbly, with no appetite. I was stunned at my reaction and looked inside myself. What I found was a big dark *blah*. I had little interest in Forrest or life altogether. For his sake, I tried to put a good face on our time together, but when I came home, I immediately called Rick. "Honey," I said, "I think I'm *depressed*." The light bulb went on for him too, and we had one of our best talks in years.

Because we were starting to realize that I had a real *health* problem, Rick became even more supportive. Nonetheless, we still did not know what to do, nor did the doctors we consulted. Meanwhile, my health was getting worse, not better. Soon after Laurel's second birthday, I developed chronic diarrhea, which was so serious that it sometimes called me out of bed in the middle of the night. I started to have a tremor in my hands, more intense memory problems, and a sense of "roaring" under my skin. I weaned Laurel, which helped me feel a little less drained, but nonetheless, my chronic back and shoulder pain increased further.

Then came the third breakthrough, around the time Forrest turned six. One day, while talking with a friend about how poor our diets had become since we had kids, I had a brainstorm that my pregnancies, breastfeeding, and stress might have taken something out of my body. I asked a physician to run a series of blood tests, and the results finally brought some clarity to what I'd been experiencing. All of my minerals were far below the normal range. Deficient minerals can compromise every system in the body—such as connective tissue and muscle fiber (thus my chronic back pain)—and that is exactly what happened to me. Many of my amino acids were also low, and these are the crucial building blocks of proteins that in turn make many neurochemicals, hormones, and other important things in your body.

These findings prompted me to assess my endocrine system, and there, too, I was running on empty. My hormone levels were generally at the low end of the so-called normal range. That range typically runs from roughly the 15th to 85th percentiles—or even the 5th to 95th percentiles—so that a low result at the 20th or even the 10th percentile could be considered "normal, not a problem." But "normal" on a lab report does not necessarily mean "optimal" for an individual! My doctor, a good general practitioner, reassured me that these findings were nothing to worry about, but years later, more specialized physicians concluded that my health probably would have been improved if we would have addressed my endocrine system when I was first tested.

The fourth breakthrough came some months later when a holistically oriented doctor suggested that I make sure there wasn't an infection in my digestive tract. Testing revealed that I had developed a serious case of gastrointestinal dysfunction. I had contracted digestive parasites: *Entamoeba histolytica*, one of the causes of amoebic dysentery. I had never traveled outside the country, so I must have acquired them on a stray leaf of lettuce or something similar. A healthy person's bodily defenses would probably have gobbled those parasites up and ended the invasion right there. But my vulnerable immune system was worn down by years of stress, and it was soon overrun. The results were nasty. Gastrointestinal pathogens (i.e., parasites and some bacteria and viruses) disrupt the digestive tract and impair the body's ability to absorb and make use of the nutrients in food. Some also excrete toxic substances, and these can disrupt the subtle balance of brain chemistry, thereby increasing depression, anxiety, and a sense of mental fog.

The Diagnosis

Now I finally had an accurate diagnosis: I had entered motherhood with low nutritional reserves due to years of a mediocre diet and a digestive tract that was far from optimal because of years of antibiotics and too much sugar. These reserves were drained further by several pregnancies, five years of continuous breastfeeding, and lots of hard work. The impact of maternal stress on my GI tract made it harder to absorb nutrients, so I became even more depleted. Nutrient shortages and stress had weakened my immune system and endocrine system, and gastrointestinal pathogens had exploited those vulnerabilities and infested my body. The results were digestive problems, tremor and other neurological symptoms, fatigue, muscle tension and pain, depression, and anxiety. In short, I had developed a severe case of what we came to call "depleted mother syndrome."

The Treatment

With this clarity, I was able to pursue a course of treatment that has enormously improved my health, although it took time and there were many ups and downs. Because my problems were complex and severe, I used many approaches over a number of years. It is unlikely you will need to do anything as elaborate.

In sum, I took the following actions:

- Multiple rounds of antiparasitic medications and herbs to treat the digestive pathogens
- A diet low in sweets (to stop feeding the bad microbes) and high in vegetables and protein
- A multivitamin/mineral supplement each day, as well as beneficial bacteria for my digestive tract
- Chinese herbs and acupuncture
- Iodine to support thyroid function (initially my body could not tolerate hormones given directly)
- Biofeedback for tension and tremor
- Antidepressants for low mood, insomnia, and chronic pain. I took these with some reluctance and tapered off after two years. I am now aware of more natural methods that might have been as useful, but the medications were an effective

bridge to healthier functioning, and they gave me a clearer head with which to make decisions about my overall care.

These days I can still get thrown off by overstress or poor nutrition (such as sugar binges over the holidays—alas), but now I usually have decent energy, normal digestive functioning, no pain, no tremors, and a positive mood. I feel very grateful that the methods worked.

In retrospect, though, probably the most useful intervention of all was intangible: By acquiring a greater understanding of maternal health, I was able to make sense out of all the changes in my body and come up with a realistic plan that succeeded in helping me feel a whole lot better. Knowledge about your health gives you choices and a sense of direction, which is why there's so much detail in this chapter. Feel

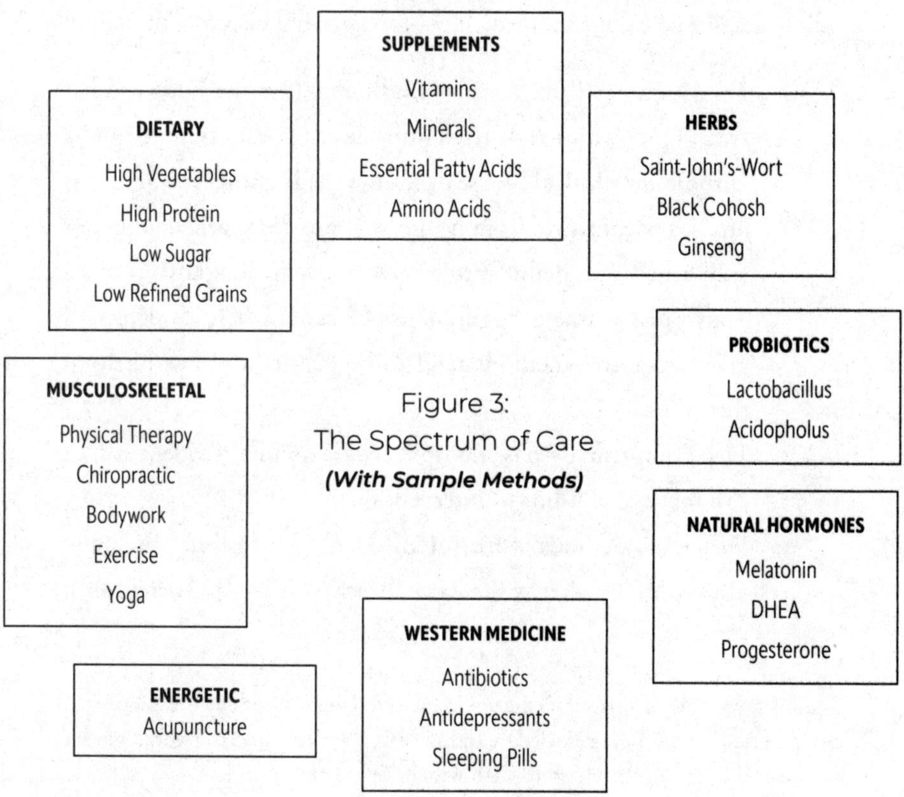

Figure 3:
The Spectrum of Care
(With Sample Methods)

free to skim the parts that don't seem relevant to you, and talk with supportive professionals about the parts that do.

THE SPECTRUM OF CARE

In our experience, the best way to replenish and settle your body is generally to combine conventional medicine with sensible complementary methods, all resting on the foundation of basic wellness practices described in chapter 4. This integrated approach is increasingly accepted, and its methods form a spectrum of care that includes energetic, musculoskeletal, dietary, nutritional supplementation, probiotic, natural hormonal, and conventional medical approaches.*

There are many advantages in considering this whole spectrum of care—not just conventional medicine—for reversing maternal depletion:

- Depletion has three features that integrative methods excel at treating: nutritional deficits, imbalanced bodily systems, and a chronic, subclinical course over time ("sub-clinical" conditions are clear departures from health that are not severe enough, or sufficiently well defined, to receive a specific diagnosis).
- Your body is like a fragile house of cards when it's depleted, and integrative methods tend to be gentler and less likely to disturb it.
- Depletion usually has multiple causes and consequences that call for several kinds of interventions.
- Different methods work for different people, but you don't always know what will succeed until you try it. Therefore, if

* Additions to the spectrum of care could include Ayurvedic medicine, homeopathy, and traditional practices used by Indigenous people around the world, but we are focusing here on the methods with which we are most familiar.

you come at a problem with several approaches, if one doesn't help, chances are that another will.

- Different types of interventions often work together synergistically, so that the whole is greater than the sum of the parts.
- A comprehensive approach brings together professionals with different perspectives, which means a check on each other's assumptions.
- The spectrum of care gives you multiple options, so you can choose the ones that feel best to you; for instance, you could want to treat a depressed mood with antidepressants, or you might prefer first trying regular exercise.

In sum, we recommend that your health care start with a physician in order to rule out or treat any serious medical condition. But we also suggest that it does not end there, because of the benefits that are potentially available to you in integrative methods. Individually, many of those gains will be mild, but when you start adding them up, mild + mild + mild + mild + mild = major improvement in your health and well-being.

A conventional physician may not be familiar with the integrative approaches we describe, and in some cases might try to talk you out of them. Much the same could be said for some alternative practitioners with regard to conventional medicine. We think any intervention for your health should be judged on its merits, not tradition or dogma. For guidance in discerning the strengths and weaknesses of different approaches, finding competent professionals who understand the spectrum of care, and getting the most out of any assessment, please be sure to look at Appendix D.

As you look at the options within the spectrum of care in the rest of this chapter, please don't be overwhelmed at all the possibilities: The point is that there are *lots* of things that could help you feel better if you've become depleted. Just knowing that there are things you can do can improve your sense of well-being, especially if you feel at all worn down or dispirited. It probably took some time for you to become depleted, and it will take a while to turn that around. It's more important to keep plugging away at a broad and sensible effort to replenish and settle your body than to seek one hypothetical magic bullet that might make everything better.

So let's get down to business, starting with the primary pathway to replenishing your body, the gastrointestinal system.

YOUR GASTROINTESTINAL SYSTEM

If your gastrointestinal system—housed mainly in the stomach and intestines—is not in good working order, you will get fewer of the nutrients you need to handle all the demands and stresses that come with being a mother. That means you need to take care of three important elements:

- **Membranes:** The surface area of your small intestine could cover the floor of a typical studio apartment if all the millions of microscopic folds in its walls were laid out flat. This forms a membrane between the contents of the digestive tract and the rest of the body that absorbs food and filters out damaging substances.
- **Enzymes and digestive acids:** Enzymes in your mouth start the process of digestion, and then hydrochloric acid in the stomach breaks food down further. Enzymes secreted into the upper end of the small intestine cut these particles into even smaller pieces, and then they are absorbed in the small and large intestine.
- **Microbial ecology:** Modern science is only beginning to understand the effects of the microbiome, vast populations

of microorganisms living in your intestines. These include hundreds of species of bacteria—some benign and some harmful—as well as viruses, yeast, and perhaps some single-celled parasites. The beneficial microflora aid digestion, make essential vitamins, and keep harmful microbes in check.

What Can Disturb the Gastrointestinal System

The GI system is easily disturbed by stress—and that's part of a mother's daily diet! As we saw in chapter 1, stress causes the mouth to produce less saliva and the stomach to secrete less hydrochloric acid. It also leads the small intestine to reduce necessary contractions, and decreases blood flow to the stomach and intestines. If the demands of raising a family give a mom more headaches, increased use of nonsteroidal anti-inflammatory drugs (NSAIDs), such as aspirin or ibuprofen, can irritate and inflame the lining of the gut. Nutritional shortages, accumulating over several years, may deplete the intestinal walls of the "bricks and mortar" that keep them in tip-top shape. In order for digestion to proceed properly, things have to keep moving along, but pregnancy often makes the GI system sluggish, and the effects can linger after the baby is born if your diet is not optimal.

Maternal stress can disrupt the delicate balance of the microbial ecology in the digestive tract, leading to a condition termed *dysbiosis*. In addition, a mother's reliance on quick and ultraprocessed foods—which usually contain lots of white flour and sugar—can foster a population explosion of various microorganisms (especially if her immune system is already taxed), worsening the dysbiosis. It's like a lawn: A few weeds are inconspicuous and easy to pull, but if the crabgrass takes over, it damages the whole yard, and it's really hard to remove. Dysbiosis has been linked to numerous GI symptoms, including constipation, diarrhea, cramping, and inflammation in the digestive tract, as well as to autoimmune conditions and other disruptions of overall health.

Further, these factors may, in turn, lead to what is called a food sensitivity, in which the immune system "thinks" there is something threatening about a particular food and keeps producing high levels of antibodies to it. Why would this happen? When your GI system is disturbed, the membranes of the digestive tract may become inflamed and compromised, allowing food molecules that have been incompletely broken down to pass through into the bloodstream; this condition is termed *intestinal permeability*, or "leaky gut syndrome." The sentinels of the immune system know what a thoroughly digested bit of bread is supposed to look like, but these oversized, partially processed "macromolecules" could be a threat, so the body's defenses are mobilized to protect you, and an antibody to a particular food is formed that triggers an immune reaction the next time you eat it.

In a vicious cycle, a food sensitivity can prompt the immune system to attack that food in your digestive tract, which creates more inflammation and makes it even easier for incompletely digested food particles to enter your bloodstream, leading to more sensitivities. Clearly, it pays to keep the GI system humming along at peak efficiency, fully digesting the foods that come down the hatch.

The effects of motherhood on the endocrine, nervous, and immune systems can indirectly impact the GI system. For example, irregularities in thyroid hormones (more likely after children) can lead to constipation (low thyroid) or diarrhea (high thyroid). Disturbances in neurotransmitters such as serotonin can trouble your digestive tract. If the immune system is weakened by maternal stress, it is less able to protect the digestive tract against infection.

Of course, factors unrelated to motherhood could also impact your gastrointestinal system, like work stress or overuse of laxatives. Therefore, we suggest that you discuss any GI symptoms with your doctor. (This point applies, as well, to the nervous, endocrine, and immune systems.)

Signs and Symptoms of Disturbance in the GI System

In our experience, many mothers have some kind of disturbance in their gastrointestinal systems. You might experience indigestion, a feeling of overfullness or gassiness after eating that may include heartburn. There could be pain in your stomach, intestinal cramping, or a general sense of discomfort throughout your abdomen. Or nausea, constipation, diarrhea, or gas. Any one of these symptoms feels bad, plus it makes it harder to give your full attention to your children or work.

GI system dysregulation can also lead to problems in other parts of the body. Poor absorption in the digestive tract causes shortages of nutrients elsewhere. More speculatively, some evidence suggests that food sensitivities can lead to an overactive immune system in general, which would tend to increase inflammation as well as mucus (and nondraining mucus is a too-friendly medium for bacterial growth). Many holistically oriented practitioners, including Jan, have noted an apparent association between vaginal yeast infections and an overgrowth of yeast in the digestive tract.* And the toxins excreted by pathogenic microbes may lead to fatigue, inflammation, depressed mood, or poor memory.

* Low levels of yeast are normally present in the digestive tract, usually without apparent harm. Yet high levels, particularly in terms of your own body and its needs, can cause diarrhea, increase the likelihood of vaginal infections, and produce microtoxins that can weaken your immune system. Additionally, in our experience, when populations of intestinal yeast are reduced, there is usually an improvement in energy and overall well-being.

Gastrointestinal Assessment

The first consideration in gastrointestinal assessment is evaluating whether there is an illness, such as an ulcer, inflammatory bowel disease, or cancer. To find out, start with your doctor, who may refer you to a specialist called a gastroenterologist. And when you assess *any* system of your body, it is important to rule out other possible causes of health problems. For example, fatigue could be due to nutritional depletion—but it could also be a result of thyroid disease, autoimmune disorders, anemia, malnutrition, alcohol abuse, or chronic fatigue syndrome.

Next, you could pursue innovative and specialized laboratory testing (which, alas, may not be covered by your insurance). Unless your doctor focuses on nutritional medicine or holistic health, he or she may be unfamiliar with or even dismissive of these tests. In order to find a professional who is, see Appendix D.

You can find out if there are any shortages of key nutrients through analyzing your blood or urine, and your symptoms will guide the focus of testing. For example, dry skin and hair suggest a look at essential fatty acids, while fatigue, shortness of breath, or a pale complexion may be due to insufficient iron. Amino acids can be assessed through a urine or blood sample; we encourage many mothers to do this since amino acids are so often depleted in them. While an iron panel is a routine test, other minerals—as well as vitamins and essential fatty acids—require a specialized assessment. Multiple deficits may point to overall GI dysfunction, especially if you have a reasonably good diet and take a multivitamin/mineral supplement.

Pathogenic intestinal microorganisms—such as parasites and certain bacteria—can be assessed through stool tests, which can also reveal unhealthily high levels of yeast. A breath test is used to find small intestinal bacterial overgrowth (SIBO). A urine test for organic acids can provide a useful snapshot of the by-products of these tiny organisms; it is particularly helpful in assessing anaerobic bacteria that are nearly impossible to detect in a stool test (since they die on contact with oxygen). Finally, beneficial bacteria can be assessed to see if there are sufficient quantities of these helpful bugs in your digestive tract.

Allergies and food sensitivities are assessed through skin and blood tests and elimination diets. Skin tests detect foods (and other substances, like airborne molds) that you have an immediate, strong reaction to—such as getting hives after eating shellfish. Blood tests measuring the immunoglobulin G (IgG) antibody can identify responses to foods that build up more slowly. Because your immune system reacts to food in multiple ways, no one test is perfect, and arguably the most useful way to decide if you are sensitive to a food is to eliminate it for at least a week and perhaps longer and observe the results. You could also keep a daily diary of what you eat and any symptoms; sometimes, when you look back at what you've recorded, you can see some patterns.

In general, any one of the tests above may miss a genuine problem (called a "false-negative" error; see Appendix D for more on this error). If you have GI symptoms but a test doesn't seem to identify a specific cause, keep persisting and looking at your gastrointestinal system from different angles, perhaps with other professionals. Meanwhile, you could intervene cautiously, even without clear assessment findings, using methods in the spectrum of care that have little chance of harm, such as energetic, dietary, or probiotic.

Balancing Your Gastrointestinal System

Much like it's good to have variety in the foods you can eat, it's good that there are so many things you can do to improve the functioning of your GI system.

Energetic. Promoting gastrointestinal health has long been a cornerstone of traditional Chinese medicine, and there is evidence that acupuncture could help balance your GI system, including by stimulating peristalsis (the contractions in the intestines that move food and waste products along).

Musculoskeletal. One surprisingly simple way to reduce the effects of stress on the digestive tract is to do a minute or so of slow deep breathing before meals, which will tend to engage the parasympathetic branch of your nervous system and calm your body. If your child is old enough, see if you can get her to join you—and maybe she'll be more willing to eat her peas!

Dietary. On the foundation of the nutritional approach described in the previous chapter, consider these additional suggestions:

- **Sugar:** If you know or suspect that dysbiosis is an issue, you may be able to reduce problematic microbes by eliminating sugar, refined carbohydrates, and alcohol (which converts quickly to sugars); because of the high sugar content in fruit, you shouldn't have more than two pieces a day. Once the coast is clear—indicated by an end to symptoms as well as laboratory testing—you can usually return to the sugar guidelines in chapter 4.
- **Fiber:** Try to consume about 25 grams of fiber each day. In part because fiber-rich foods often require more preparation time, mothers tend to eat too few of them, but fiber both aids the movement of food through the digestive tract and supports beneficial bacteria. High-fiber foods include whole grains, legumes, beans, many fruits (especially pears and apples), and various vegetables. You could make a big pot of rich soup (split pea, lentil, bean, etc.)—see the Happy, Healthy Mom stew in chapter 4, as a big help in both getting enough fiber and eating well. If you can't get your daily dose of fiber from foods alone, you can take it as a supplement, but

then be sure to drink at least 8 cups of water a day—which is good for your health, anyway.

- **Food sensitivities:** Many people have GI reactions to certain foods, particularly gluten, dairy products (though butter and sometimes cream may be tolerable), corn, eggs, soy, and chocolate (sorry . . .). Eat as few foods as possible to which you are sensitive. Jan has had many patients who experienced dramatic improvement in their digestive tracts by eliminating offending foods. If you have any GI symptoms, try eating no gluten or dairy products for a couple of weeks, and you might be amazed by the results. A mild sensitivity can often be managed by eating a food only once every few days, but a moderate to severe sensitivity usually calls for total elimination for at least 6 months. Sometimes it is possible to reintroduce the food sparingly into your diet, but often it will remain something that you'll never do well with. Numerous cookbooks are available with delicious recipes for foods that can replace the ones that disturb your digestion. Diet is largely a matter of habit. After getting through the phase of withdrawal and shifting the habit to other foods, you could be quite content with your new diet, especially with the rewards of feeling so much better.
- **SIBO (small intestinal bacterial overgrowth):** If you've tried standard, well-intended recommendations for lots of fiber and whole grains, and found that they're not improving your GI issues or even making them worse, you may have SIBO. SIBO is a common underlying cause of irritable bowel syndrome, and it must be dealt with in a particular way.

SIBO develops from poor movement of food in the small intestine, most often due to an incident of food poisoning or occasionally from some scar tissue adhesions, such as after surgery. When the food you eat is not moving properly, populations of problematic bacteria increase. Then when foods, especially carbohydrates, enter the small intestine, they feed these bacteria, producing significant amounts of gases in the process. Depending upon what type of gas this is, one might experience painful bloating and either diarrhea or constipation.

If you find that you are getting bloated around 30 minutes to 2 hours after a meal with lots of carbohydrates, that could be a sign you have SIBO, and you should investigate this possibility. A breath test is the main way to formally diagnose SIBO.

The discovery of SIBO has changed the way physicians and other practitioners have thought about irritable bowel syndrome. What once was thought of as a stress response is now understood as having biological underpinnings. Irritable bowel can cause lots of discomfort and pain, so it is worthwhile to understand it and seek treatment.

Although a comprehensive treatment for SIBO exceeds the scope of this book, these are the fundamental aspects:

1. Avoid foods that particularly feed the bacteria in the small intestine. This mostly involves minimizing carbohydrates, since proteins and fats are not major food sources for these bacteria. This approach is called the low-FODMAP diet because it avoids a group of short-chain carbohydrates that are Fermentable Oligosaccharides, Disaccharides, Monosaccharides, And Polyols. See the box for a list of major FODMAP foods to avoid. A common approach involves eliminating all FODMAP foods until SIBO symptoms improve; then you could gradually reintroduce them one at a time to see which ones trigger your specific symptoms.
2. Kill the overgrowth of bacteria in the upper small intestine with prescription antibiotics or an herbal antimicrobial. This approach requires the involvement of your health care provider.

3. Increase the motility of the small intestine. It is possible to do this with some drugs and also some herbal products. If poor motility is caused by scar tissue, you may be able to improve this with osteopathic visceral bodywork.

Common High-FODMAP Foods to Avoid or Limit

Fruits: Apples, pears, mangoes, cherries, watermelon
Vegetables: Onions, garlic, cauliflower, broccoli, asparagus
Legumes: Lentils, chickpeas, kidney beans, most legumes
Dairy: Anything with lactose, including milk, soft cheeses, yogurt
The gluten grains: Wheat, rye, barley, some oats
Sweeteners: Honey, high-fructose corn syrup, sugar
Other: Certain processed foods with FODMAP-containing additives such as sugar alcohols (sorbitol, mannitol, maltitol, or xylitol), gums (guar and xanthan), and starches (potato, tapioca, etc.)

Supplements. Taking the MSDV (see Appendix C) of nutrients can help support your GI system (as well as other systems), especially if there is a shortage of a key nutrient in your body. For example, essential fatty acids are needed for the walls of your intestines, plus they may help with serious GI disturbances, such as ulcerative colitis. Going one step further, doses above the MSDV—what we call the intensive daily dose (IDD)—of one or more of the nutrients on the next page may be able to provide additional benefit to a gastrointestinal tract that's been disturbed by the stresses and demands of motherhood, particularly if there is a functional deficiency in that nutrient. While some studies and practitioners have found benefits in even higher doses, we generally suggest that you not go beyond our IDDs unless you are working with a licensed professional who has experience in doing so. All of the IDDs are summarized in Appendix C.

Nutrient	Intensive Daily Dose (IDD)
Vitamin C	2 grams up to "bowel tolerance" (the maximum dose that does not lead to diarrhea), divided into at least two separate doses, and buffered if you have an ulcer or experience stomach irritation
Vitamin E	800 IU (use a product that has a high level of gamma-tocopherol)
Zinc	30 mg
L-glutamine	1–10 grams
Essential fatty acids	2,000–4,000 mg of omega-3 fish oil containing equal parts DHA and EPA

To mobilize the enzymes in your GI system, follow the classic advice to chew your food well. Yes, sometimes you've got only 8 minutes for lunch, but whenever you can, take your time between bites—at least enough to set your fork down. And drink liquids in moderation during meals—especially if they're cold (which reduces blood flow to your digestive tract)—so as not to dilute your enzymes.

Taking digestive enzymes as supplements may also be helpful in general, as well as lower your chance of developing a food sensitivity. There are two types: plant- and animal-based. Generally, plant enzymes are taken at the beginning of a meal, based on the theory that they are more able to survive the acid in the stomach, while animal-derived enzymes are typically taken at the end; for dosages and other details, look at the label on the bottle.

Herbs. Many Chinese herbal formulas "tonify the spleen qi," metaphorical shorthand for strengthening the digestive tract. Two formulas mentioned in chapter 4 may be particularly beneficial. Bu zhong yi qi tang is believed to strengthen the digestive tract and immune system, and we've seen dan zhi xiao yao san be useful for individuals whose digestive tracts are especially vulnerable to becoming disturbed by stress. Each formula is meant to be used over several months, rather than as a quick fix. They can be purchased online from Chinese herb pharmacies or from an acupuncturist, who can also make a customized formula to tonify your digestive tract.

Many Western herbs might also benefit your GI system. For stomach pain, licorice root—only in the form of deglycyrrhizinated licorice (DGL)—has a soothing effect, and studies suggest that it can reduce gastric pain and even help heal ulcers. Typical dosage range from 250 to 750 mg, taken up to three times a day. For overgrowth of microbes in the small or large intestines, several herbs can help reduce these populations, including garlic, goldenseal, and oregano (this last herb is best used when it is emulsified or enteric coated).

With mild GI system symptoms, you could try one of these Western herbs on your own for a month or so and see if they give you some relief. It's generally best to start at the low end of the range of dosing given on the label and increase gradually, if at all. Sometimes a "die off" reaction can occur in which symptoms get worse for a few days—presumably because the microbes are releasing toxins as they die. If you have a strong reaction to the herbs, your symptoms are moderate to severe to start with, or the herbs don't help much—please seek out the care of an experienced practitioner. During and after you've finished a trial of antimicrobial herbs, you should supplement with probiotics (see below) to increase good populations of beneficial bacteria (i.e., first kill the bad guys, then reinforce the good guys).

Probiotics. These beneficial microorganisms crowd out pathogenic ones as well as aid digestion in general. Lactobacillus bacteria (such as acidophilus) occur naturally in yogurt, but you can also get a much more concentrated supply of probiotics in supplements from a health food store, including lactobacillus strains and bifidobacteria (such as bifidus). Some strains may be more effective than others; for example, lactobacillus GG has been clearly shown to decrease GI infection. Probiotics should be refrigerated both in the store and after you bring them home, and check for a guarantee of viable organisms on the label of the bottle. There are several schools of thought about the best time to take probiotics, but in general, we suggest you do so between meals.

Conventional medicine. As we've said, if your GI system is disturbed, you should tell your doctor, who may refer you to a specialist. The treatment options include antidiarrheal agents, antispasmodics, and low doses of antidepressants. You could also try over-the-counter drugs for indigestion, constipation, and diarrhea. But these interventions are aimed at reducing symptoms or treating a specific condition, not at replenishing and balancing bodily systems as a whole—and those are your primary goals when you are reversing depletion. While Pepto-Bismol or a laxative might give you temporary relief, the underlying causes of a disturbed GI system will persist unless you care for the system in general by reducing your stress, following general wellness practices, and exploring the options we've described.

For instance, consider the use of antibiotics to treat a bacterial or parasitic infection in your digestive tract. These are a double-edged sword, attacking a specific pathogen while disturbing your GI system in general. If an infection is not yet deeply entrenched—let's say you just returned from a trip overseas, but some microbes have unfortunately hitched a ride back with you—then antibiotics could be a silver bullet. But we have known numerous people, including Jan, for whom one or more rounds of antibiotics were unsuccessful in eradicating their intestinal pathogens. For this reason, some professionals use a combination of drugs and herbs, since the herbs (though less potent) can be tolerated for much longer periods of time. And in order to address your gastrointestinal system as a whole, you should also starve the pathogens (by eliminating sugar and refined flour products), compete with them by adding probiotics, and repair their damage to the linings of the digestive tract with EFAs and L-glutamine. It's sobering to realize that microbes have had a three-billion-year evolutionary head start over multicellular organisms like ourselves. They are tough adversaries, and we suggest you work with a professional who is experienced in using an integrated approach in their treatment.

YOUR NERVOUS SYSTEM

Let's start with a little experiment. Think about your child giving you a hug, and imagine the emotions and body sensations you'd feel. Now, let all that go, and try thinking about her fussing at you, and imagine your emotions and body sensations.

In each case, whatever you felt involved the workings of your nervous system. From the most subtle appreciation of a little flower to the most intense rage, from a cheerful mood to a heavy cloud that smothers the life out of a moment that by every reason should be happy—your moment-to-moment stream of consciousness is based on underlying neural structures and processes.

To accomplish this extraordinary feat, your brain has about 85 billion neurons amid another 100 billion or so support cells. On average, a neuron will connect with several thousand other neurons at junctions called *synapses*, where one neuron is almost touching another one. This makes a complex network inside your head with over 100 trillion nodes, each like a little microprocessor. A primary form of neural activity involves releasing chemical messengers called *neurotransmitters* (for simplicity, we are using this term broadly) across these tiny synaptic gaps. A typical neuron can fire 10 to 100 times per second, which means that over a trillion or so synaptic events involving neurotransmitters could have occurred in your brain . . . in the time it took you to read this sentence.

So you can see why neurotransmitters are so important. In order for you to feel good—or to have anything function very effectively in your body—the system of neurotransmitters must be in top working order. Of course, so must the rest of the brain. Because the nervous system contains such complexity, we'll focus mainly on neurotransmitters. And within that aspect of the nervous system, our emphasis will be on the factors that affect emotional well-being, since anxiety, frustration, and depressed mood are so common among mothers.

What Can Disturb the Nervous System

Of all the bodily systems, the nervous system is the one in which there is the most intimate connection between physiology and lived experience. The effects of motherhood on your body can send ripples—sometimes shock waves—through your brain and thus your mind:

- **Stress:** Whether you're intervening in sibling quarrels or worrying about a sick child, those everyday stresses of raising children can change the balance of neurotransmitters in your brain and cause depressed mood and poorer concentration and memory.
- **Nutrition:** Your outflow of nutrients (due to pregnancy, breastfeeding, and the work and stress of raising a family) can lead to deficits in substances that either are neurotransmitters—such as the amino acids taurine, glycine, and GABA—or are needed to build them. For example, taurine has calming and soothing effects, but as mentioned in chapter 4, there's a high demand for it during breastfeeding, and without an excellent diet, it can be lacking in a mother's body.
- **Other bodily systems:** Bearing and rearing children can affect your brain indirectly through their impacts on other systems in your body. In the endocrine system, decreases or fluctuations

in estrogen or progesterone—whether following childbirth or due to chronic stress—can impact several neurotransmitter systems, leading to depression, anxiety, or a poorer memory. Thyroid dysregulation after childbirth or due to an autoimmune condition related to motherhood can lead to depression. And as cortisol rises due to stress, DHEA tends to decline, which has been linked to depressed mood.

In the immune system, allergies and inflammation (which often increase after having children) can lower your mood. Gastrointestinal dysfunction due to maternal stress can impair the absorption of nutrients needed to make serotonin and other neurochemicals.

Signs and Symptoms of Disturbances in Neurotransmitters

Fleeting, everyday experiences of sadness, fatigue, or anxiety do not in themselves suggest a fundamental change in your brain chemistry. But chronic experiences of this sort just might. For example, consider the effects of disturbances in these neurotransmitter systems:

- Serotonin: Depression, irritability, anxiety, insomnia, rumination
- Norepinephrine: Depression and fatigue
- Dopamine: Depression and fatigue
- GABA (gamma-aminobutyric acid): Anxiety and insomnia

Brain chemistry is intimately involved in your fundamental sense of "me," and it can be very troubling to experience an unpleasant change within your own mind, like finding a crack in the walls of the innermost sanctum of your castle. Happily, you can get a good assessment of what is happening in your nervous system, and there are many effective things you can do to replenish and balance it.

Assessment of Neurotransmitters

There are two levels to assessing neurotransmitters: your subjective experience (symptoms) and their objective status in your body (signs). For example, most evaluations for depression—and prescriptions for antidepressants—are based on the first level alone, using questions such as: *How long have you felt this way? How frequently, within a typical week? How intense does it get?* Additionally, laboratory tests through your health care providers can reveal shortfalls in amino acids that function as (or like) neurotransmitters, or in vitamins and minerals needed to build neurotransmitters. Other tests can measure the breakdown products of serotonin, dopamine, and norepinephrine—like estimating how many animals live in a meadow by counting their scat.

Balancing the Neurotransmitters of Mood

Our emphasis here is on balancing neurotransmitters in general in order to lift your mood, rather than treating any specific psychological condition, such as depression. If you have moderate to severe depression, these methods might help some, but they will probably not resolve it completely, and you should be sure to see a therapist or doctor. (Also see the section on depression in chapter 3.)

Energetic. Studies have shown that acupuncture can lift depressed mood.

Musculoskeletal. Regular exercise can help lift depressed mood, sometimes working as well as an antidepressant.

Dietary. Since shortages of specific nutrients can affect how you feel, it's important to eat nourishing, well-rounded meals. Be careful about a low-protein diet if you tend toward a depressed mood, since that would reduce amino acids needed for healthy brain chemistry.

Additionally, one food that can lower your mood when consumed in excess is sugar. Studies have found that eliminating sugar can improve mood. Eliminating alcohol could help as well.

Supplements. Studies have shown that deficits in the nutrients listed in the chart—especially omega-3 essential fatty acids and vitamin B6—are associated with depressed mood. For example, shortages in B6 reduce the conversion of tryptophan into serotonin. Supplementation with the intensive daily doses shown in the chart, especially when there is a deficiency in those nutrients, could help lift your spirits. (Tip: Add individual B-vitamins only if you are already consuming MSDV levels of B-vitamins in general.)

Nutrient	Intensive Daily Dose (IDD)
Omega-3 oils	2,000–4,000 mg fish oil (with equal parts DHA and EPA)
Vitamin B6	50 mg pyridoxal-5-phosphate (the active form of B6)
Vitamin B12	Try sublingual tablets, 2,000 mcg, 1–3/day; severe deficiencies may require B12 injections
Folic acid	800 mcg; use a methylated folic acid
Iron	If lab testing shows deficiency, 30 mg twice daily between meals; a good form is iron bisglycinate, which causes minimal digestive issues; try to avoid taking iron at the same time as calcium since one reduces the absorption of the other
Zinc	30 mg
Magnesium	400–800 mg, ideally as magnesium glycinate; decrease if there is soft stool or diarrhea; if you are constipated, try magnesium citrate

Amino acids also play an important role in your mood, and supplementing one could lift your spirits if it is deficient in your body and the neurotransmitter it supports is the principal source of the slump in your mood. In general, because your body already has normal pathways for metabolizing and eliminating amino acids—unlike medications or herbs—there tend to be few if any side effects.

Tryptophan is used to make serotonin, and some studies have shown that supplementing it or *5-hydroxytryptophan* (5-HTP, a metabolite of tryptophan that is one step closer to serotonin) may be successful in the treatment of mild depression. For suggestions about taking tryptophan, please see the previous chapter. Although the dosage of 5-HTP commonly used in studies of depression is 200–300 mg/day, we recommend starting at 50 mg and then increasing by 50 mg every few days, depending on how you feel. Do not exceed 200 mg per day, and do not take 5-HTP along with Saint-John's-wort, antidepressants (especially MAO inhibitors), or any psychoactive drug or herb, unless you are doing so under an experienced practitioner's supervision.

Tyrosine is the chemical basis for the neurotransmitters norepinephrine and dopamine, which are involved in the regulation of mood. If you are deficient in tyrosine or its amino acid precursor, phenylalanine, supplementing one of these may help improve your mood. A commonly used dose of either tyrosine or phenylalanine is 500–1,000 mg, and it's best taken in the morning, on an empty stomach, for good absorption and to avoid insomnia. Another amino acid, *taurine*, may have a mild calming effect and help ease irritability or tension by supporting a balanced nervous system. You could try 500 mg, taken in the morning, and to optimize its effect, make sure you're also taking at least 400 mg/day of magnesium.

Methionine is an amino acid that becomes S-adenosyl methionine (SAMe), which in turn helps the body with a process called *methylation* that is required for the production of many neurotransmitters. Low levels of SAMe are associated with depressed mood, and several well-controlled studies have found that supplementing SAMe is often quite effective in relieving depression (and it also seems helpful for joint pain). The most commonly used daily dosage of SAMe is 400–800 mg, and it should be taken in special enterically coated capsules on an empty stomach. We suggest starting at 200 mg—especially if you are sensitive to medications—or at 100 mg if you have a history of panic attacks; a person with bipolar disorder should take SAMe only under medical supervision. Also be sure you're getting the MSDV of vitamins B6 and B12, as well as folic acid. SAMe metabolizes into homocysteine, a compound linked to cardiovascular disease, and these B-vitamins help convert homocysteine into benign substances in your body.

Herbs. The most common herbal treatment for depression is *Hypericum perforatum*, also known as Saint-John's-wort. Studies have found it to be often helpful for mild depression, though it does not appear to be an effective treatment for severe depression. The dosage used is commonly 900 mg per day of "standardized extract" (containing 0.3 percent hypericin, one of the active ingredients), divided over two or three doses. Although some people may feel it in the first few days, it often takes several weeks for the full effects to be apparent.

As with any herb you take, use Saint-John's-wort that is produced by a reputable botanical company to ensure that you are getting both high quality and the correct dosage. About 2 to 20 percent of people taking Saint-John's-wort suffer side effects (which may diminish after a few weeks), such as mild gastrointestinal disturbance, drowsiness, dizziness, or sensitivity to sunlight. Do not use Saint-John's-wort with 5-HTP, antidepressants, or any psychoactive drug or herb. If you are on *any* prescription medication—in particular, for contraception, high blood pressure, or HIV—ask your doctor before trying Saint-John's-wort as it can reduce the effectiveness of other medications.

Hormones. From a practical standpoint, hormones come in three varieties:

- **Natural or bioidentical, available over the counter:** Whether they are extracted from natural sources or manufactured, these hormones are identical to their form in your body (e.g., melatonin, DHEA,* progesterone).
- **Natural or bioidentical, available by prescription only:** These include thyroid, testosterone, and estrogen.
- **Manufactured, modified versions of the hormone, available by prescription only:** These molecules are similar but not identical to the hormones in your body and have hormone-like effects. Examples include progestins such as Provera. They are commonly found in birth control pills.

The natural hormone—the one your body is adapted to—generally has advantages over a near copy, though there may be specific circumstances in which your doctor recommends the manufactured version. But beware: The fact that you can walk into your local drugstore or health food store and buy several kinds of natural hormones may give the impression that there's little to worry about, yet just because something is "natural" or available without a prescription doesn't mean it's harmless. Hormones are powerful substances, so we must repeat this point: You should *always* consult with a licensed health care practitioner about their use—and especially if you are pregnant or breastfeeding.

Supplementing DHEA may help lift a depressed mood, particularly if there is an adrenal insufficiency (you can find out by testing

* Technically, DHEA is often not considered a hormone since there are no receptor sites for it specifically. But it is a crucial building block for many other hormones, and for simplicity, we will discuss it as if it were a hormone.

as you'll see later on), and may increase sex drive. But there are also risks in supplementing with DHEA, since it is the basis for numerous hormones, including estrogen and testosterone, and unnaturally high levels in those hormones can be problematic. We suggest you discuss the pros and cons with your doctor before trying DHEA.

Conventional medicine. Antidepressant medications are one of the great medical success stories in the last century, and millions of people have used them to good effect (including Jan). They are most often prescribed by physicians in general practice; if the first choice works for you, fine, but if not, we suggest you consult with a psychiatrist who specializes in these medicines.

Compared to the natural alternatives such as 5-HTP, antidepressants are stronger and more likely to help with moderate to severe depression. On the other hand, they are also more likely to have significant side effects, including emotional blunting, dry mouth, loss of libido, weight gain, or inability to climax. (Pregnant or breastfeeding women need to be particularly careful about the use of antidepressants.) Plus, they don't always work: They're unsuccessful about a third of the time or more, either because of a lack of efficacy or intolerable side effects. One strategy is to start with a natural remedy, and if that is not powerful enough, consider moving on to an antidepressant.

If the root cause of feeling blue is purely physiological, a biochemical intervention—such as Saint-John's-wort or Prozac—may be all you need. But if a depressed mood is due at least in part to psychological, interpersonal, or circumstantial (e.g., sleep deprivation) factors, a purely physical intervention could allow the real causes of your suffering to remain unchecked, as well as rob you of an opportunity for learning and personal growth. In many cases, biochemical approaches are best used as a short-term intervention to lift a smothering cloud and thereby free a person up to take action—in her mind, relationships, and circumstances—to improve her health and well-being over the long run.

YOUR ENDOCRINE SYSTEM

Similar to a multitasking mother, hormones manage a wide range of vital business, from the essentials of bodily survival to keeping a smile on your face. You hear so much about estrogen and progesterone because of their role in menstruation and menopause, but there are many other hormones involved in every bodily system and function, including reproduction, digestion, sleep, physical development, emotion, and thought. They travel around the body like little boats with messages, launched by various glands—such as the ovaries, pituitary, hypothalamus, or adrenals—and carried by the tides of blood and other fluids, and then docking at their destination in receptor sites perfectly designed for the shape of their hull.

Sometimes a hormone goes off to work on an organ, such as estrogen and progesterone preparing the uterine lining to play loving hostess to the embryo. Other times, the destination of a hormone is the brain itself; as a result, hormones affect memory, self-control, and mood. And sometimes the target organ is another endocrine gland—such as when the pituitary sends a message to your adrenals to secrete cortisol to handle a new stressor. Hormones affect each other in intricate feedback loops of extraordinary complexity and dynamism. Some even turn into other hormones, such as progesterone to cortisol. Adding a further layer of complication, one hormone may have many functions; for instance, estrogen plays an important role in memory and in promoting rapid immune responses to invading microbes. Science is learning more every day about our hormones, but there is still a lot that is not yet understood about this marvelous system.

For the endocrine system to function well, several kinds of things have to work properly:

- Correct amounts of hormones: For example, too little thyroid leads to lethargy and too much may lead to the protruding eyes and speedy buzz of Graves' disease.
- Sufficient numbers of correctly formed and available receptors that can receive the hormones circulating in your body.
- A well-regulated system: Small changes in the proportion of one hormone to another can make a very large difference. For example, it is the changing ratio of estrogen and progesterone—not their absolute quantities—that is an important factor in determining whether you'll suffer from PMS.
- Effective detoxification of the waste products of hormone metabolism so they do not accumulate in and harm your body.

What Can Disturb the Endocrine System

Conception, pregnancy, childbirth, breastfeeding, and the deepest instincts to nurture a child are all guided by your hormones. Whenever so many hundreds of complex and intertwining molecular processes are set in motion, it doesn't take much to disturb that dance—and leave the dancers reeling and out of place. For example:

- After a child is born, progesterone and estrogen crash with the delivery of the placenta (there goes a major hormone factory!), dropping to almost a hundredth of their previous levels. This may lead to seemingly unprovoked weepy moments, and life can feel like being caught in the spin cycle of a washing machine. Most women recover in a few weeks from the "baby blues," but progesterone and estrogen levels may end up settling down to somewhere other than an optimal point, even after the baby's first birthday.

- And of course, a new friend has moved into your home: stress. Everything from sleep disturbance to quarrels with your partner tends to rattle your progesterone, estrogen, insulin, cortisol, and thyroid hormones. On the other hand, oxytocin reduces the impact of stressors, including during the months or years in which a mother is breastfeeding.
- As for thyroid, this gland seems to be especially vulnerable during the postpartum period. One possibility is that the immune system—which has to be "turned off" in certain ways in order not to attack the developing fetus (whose DNA is different from the mother's)—may go to the other extreme in some cases when it is "turned on" after childbirth, and then start attacking the thyroid gland in an autoimmune reaction. Whatever the causes may be, the risk of thyroid problems increases several times higher after having children; about one woman in ten will develop an autoimmune disease of the thyroid gland in the postpartum period.
- Your body is designed to return to menstruation within a few months after childbirth if you are not breastfeeding, and by six months or so if you nurse. But sometimes this restoration of normal cycling does not occur smoothly, especially if you were prone to menstrual irregularities, or are now eating poorly or under a good deal of stress.
- Motherhood-related disturbance of the GI, nervous, and immune systems can also affect the endocrine system. Digestive imbalances can disturb the delicate rhythms of the hormonal dance, and deficiencies in key nutrients can weaken the dancers. The nervous system affects your hormones in part because several endocrine glands (such as the pituitary) are located within the brain; for instance, ups and downs in the neurotransmitters that regulate your mood can change your hormones as well. And disturbances

in the immune system can trigger autoimmune reactions that attack endocrine glands such as the thyroid or pancreas.

> *A . . . mother's role is to deliver children obstetrically once, and by car forever after.*
>
> Peter De Vries

Signs and Symptoms of Disturbance in the Endocrine System

Although the complexity of hormonal interaction can make it difficult to point to a single hormone as the culprit, these are some symptoms that might indicate hormonal imbalances:

- Fatigue, feeling of chilliness, low body temperature, dry skin, hair loss,* lack of menstrual periods, and a glum mood are common signs of *low thyroid.*
- Hyperactivity, racing heartbeat, tremor, bulging eyes, feeling hot, and anxiety could indicate *high thyroid.*
- Marked premenstrual symptoms of irritability, water retention, breast tenderness; irregular bleeding; or depressive feelings suggest *rapid shifts in or low levels of progesterone.*
- Hot flashes, vaginal dryness, and depressed mood could be signs of *low estrogen.*
- Waking around 4 a.m. and being unable to return to sleep, overreactions to stress, and daytime fatigue may mean *disturbed cortisol.*
- Lack of menstrual periods or continued milky discharge from the nipples may indicate *high prolactin.*

---

* Postpartum hair loss can also be a side effect of the normal drop in progesterone after birth, so ask your doctor about any significant hair loss.

- Jitters or sweating may be caused by too rapid a fall in blood sugar due to an *overproduction of insulin*.
- Low energy or mood could be a sign of *low DHEA*.

ASSESSING THE ENDOCRINE SYSTEM

There are various ways to assess your hormones. Here, we'll list only those methods most relevant to reversing depletion. General hormone assessment is typically conducted by an endocrinologist, though assessing the sex steroid hormones (estrogen, progesterone, etc.) is often done by a gynecologist.

- **Thyroid:** Thyroid testing is most commonly done through blood tests that measure thyroid stimulating hormone (TSH), which tells the thyroid gland to pump out more thyroid hormones. Blood tests can also measure two types of thyroid hormone, known as T3 and T4. High TSH is a sign that thyroid levels are low enough that the body is begging for more, while low TSH means there is too much thyroid hormone, so the gland is being asked to cut back its production. But as straightforward as this seems, there is a gray zone between high and low TSH that requires clinical judgment to consider what might be high or low for *you*. Even with seemingly "normal" levels of TSH or thyroid hormone, you may benefit from increasing the amount of active thyroid in your body through the interventions described later on.
- **Progesterone and estrogen:** These hormones can be assessed through blood and saliva tests. If a blood test is performed, your physician will make sure you take it at a particular time if you are having menstrual cycles, when progesterone and estrogen are peaking. Saliva tests are used by some practitioners who consider them to be a more sensitive measure of

the "free," unbound hormones that are actually available for use by your body. There are also panels available from some medical labs that allow you to test your hormones during the entire menstrual cycle by taking a saliva sample every three days, providing quite a clear picture of your hormonal rhythms over time.

- **Adrenal hormones:** Cortisol and DHEA levels can be tested in saliva, blood, and urine. Since there is a normal pattern of rising and falling levels of cortisol over the course of a day, this hormone is generally best assessed four times during a 24-hour period, which is easily done with saliva samples.
- **Insulin:** The glucose in your blood was probably assessed during pregnancy to make sure that you were not developing gestational diabetes. If it was high at that time, that suggests increased risk for type 2 diabetes and more reason to limit your sugar (another reason is a family history of diabetes). The standard tests for type 2 diabetes are glycated hemoglobin (HbA1c) and a fasting test of blood glucose, and other tests may be ordered by your doctor to assess the details of how your body handles sugar.

Once you have a good understanding of the current state of your hormones, you can start nudging them toward greater balance. Let's see how to address three aspects of the endocrine system that are frequently disturbed in mothers: menstruation, thyroid, and cortisol.

Balancing Your Menstrual Cycle

Menstrual imbalance often reflects a broader dysregulation in a woman's hormones. By using the spectrum of care to bring more harmony to your menstrual cycle—usually indicated by an improvement in the symptoms of PMS—you may be able to help your endocrine system in general.

First, a bit of background. PMS has many different faces—and no single solution. Its symptoms can include anxiety, depression, irritability, carbohydrate craving, or bloating—but the combination of them can vary from woman to woman, or even from month to month in the same person. The fluctuating hormones involved in these various types of PMS—such as estrogen and progesterone, and perhaps prolactin, cortisol, the androgens, or thyroid—also vary. The ways in which your body is using and metabolizing hormones probably play a role as well. Further, imbalances in various neurotransmitters have been implicated in PMS. All this complexity means that the package of interventions that will work best for you has to be individualized.

Now, some practical suggestions. Your overall well-being is the root of hormonal health, so probably the greatest improvement in your menstrual balance will come from following the wellness program in chapter 4 and decreasing your stress. Based on that foundation, let's see how you could use the spectrum of care to settle your menstrual cycle and relieve the symptoms of PMS.

Energetic. In our experience, acupuncture can sometimes be quite helpful with PMS, perhaps through its general effects on a woman's sex hormones.

Musculoskeletal. Regular exercise promotes production of carrier proteins—tugboats guiding your body's fleet of hormones—which helps keep hormone levels more even. More specifically, exercise often has a clear benefit for PMS; for example, one study showed that women who participate in sports experience less PMS than those who don't. Regular massages can help as well, either by a professional or simply swapping with your partner or a friend.

Dietary. You are likely to have less PMS if you consume less (or no) sugar, salt, refined carbohydrates, caffeine, alcohol, and dairy products, and if you increase your intake of fruits, vegetables, and other fiber-rich complex carbohydrates.

Two types of foods are worth your special attention. First, the cruciferous vegetables—particularly broccoli, Brussels sprouts, and cabbage—have a compound called indole-3-carbinol (I3C), which has been shown to affect the metabolism of estrogen in a positive way, moving it through pathways that have fewer side effects such as PMS. Second, soy foods contain phytoestrogens, molecules that are close cousins of estrogen. In the body, they seem to function like a very weak estrogen, slipping into estrogen receptors but producing a milder effect. If your estrogen levels were too high, the "competitive binding" of phytoestrogens to those receptors might gentle the impact of estrogen on your body. On the other hand, if your estrogen levels were too low, the phytoestrogens would activate some estrogen receptors, giving your body a needed boost. (This capacity of a single substance to moderate both high and low characteristics of a bodily system is termed *adaptogenic*, and it appears to be a property of several herbs, such as Siberian or *Panax* ginseng.) Of course, as with any other food or nutrient, you shouldn't consume extreme amounts such as soy with every meal. If you're not allergic to soy, you could have one serving of soy foods each day or so, and see if that helps.

Supplements. On top of a generally healthy diet—and the MSDV of essential fatty acids, vitamins, and minerals (especially calcium)—supplementing the intensive daily dose (IDD) of one or more of the following nutrients may bring greater balance to your menstrual cycle, particularly if that nutrient is lacking in your body:

Nutrient	Intensive Daily Dose (IDD) for the Menstrual Cycle
Vitamin B6	50 mg pyridoxal-5-phosphate
Vitamin E	400–800 IU; make sure gamma-tocopherol is the primary type of vitamin E
Magnesium	400–800 mg, ideally as magnesium glycinate; decrease if there is soft stool or diarrhea

Some women also seem to benefit from the essential fatty acid GLA, found in evening primrose oil or borage oil, especially for breast tenderness.

Herbs. A number of herbs or formulas may be useful for PMS. One of the most frequently used Chinese formulas for menstrual irregularities is dan zhi xiao yao san. The single herb dong quai is found in almost all Chinese formulas for women's health problems, and you can try it individually (in a 1:5 tincture, 1 teaspoon 3 times a day), although it's generally best in a formula. You could also see an acupuncturist and have a formula custom made for your individual pattern of PMS.

The western herb *Vitex agnus-castus* (chasteberry) has been shown to be helpful for PMS, but it can also reduce the effectiveness of oral contraceptives. If this is not a concern for you, you could try a standardized extract containing 0.5 percent agnuside, taking 175–225 mg/day.

Natural hormones. The research evidence is mixed for using progesterone to reduce PMS. Jan has worked with mothers who experienced symptom relief with progesterone, used either as an over-the-counter cream or as a prescription through a compounding pharmacy. If you explore this option, we recommend that you do so under the care of a licensed health care provider, and that you stop if you get uncomfortable symptoms, signaling too much progesterone.

Conventional medicine. If you try some of the suggestions above and your PMS remains moderate to severe, you might consider two options that require the care of a medical doctor. The first is oral contraceptive agents (OCAs)—aka "the pill." OCAs can impose an artificial balance on your menstrual cycle, but they also may interfere with the metabolism of some vitamins (including B6, which helps *reduce* PMS) and increase your long-term risk for heart disease, especially if you smoke or have other risk factors. Second, SSRI antidepressants such as Prozac and Lexapro—and perhaps other types of antidepressants—may relieve the depressed mood some women have with PMS, and sometimes other discomfort as well.

Balancing Thyroid Hormone

Your thyroid gland produces hormones that regulate the pace of many of the processes in your body. After children, it's more common to see thyroid levels that are too low than too high—particularly mildly to moderately low (termed *hypothyroidism*)—so that will be our focus in this section. Nonetheless, an overactive thyroid gland is a serious medical condition, and you should speak with your doctor immediately if you are concerned about that possibility.

Energetic. Some practitioners of Chinese medicine use acupuncture for hypothyroidism. If your case is mild, an energetic shift might help, but if you have moderate or severe symptoms, other forms of care will probably be required.

Supplements. Iodine combines with tyrosine to make thyroid hormone; deficits in iodine are increasingly widespread, and they can cause hypothyroidism. You could try supplementing this mineral, which is usually well assimilated in the form of kelp tablets; 150 mcg is the DV, but some practitioners go as high as 600 mcg. Or you could supplement tyrosine, which is best taken in the morning to avoid thyroid activity keeping you awake at night. You could start at 500 mg and increase the daily dose up to 1,000 mg. A third possibility would be to supplement phenylalanine, the amino acid precursor of tyrosine, which is often more easily absorbed by the body (use the same dosing as tyrosine). Supplementing tyrosine or phenylalanine is particularly worth considering if testing has found low levels of either amino acid, since they are the basis for the energizing neurotransmitters dopamine and norepinephrine (technically, when norepinephrine acts outside the nervous system, it is considered a hormone). If you try one of these three options, start with a low dose and increase it slowly, if at all, in order to avoid pushing the pendulum too far in the other direction, toward overstimulation.

Selenium and zinc help activate thyroid hormone in your body, and it's important to make sure you are getting enough. The DV of selenium is 55 mcg, and you could try up to 200–400 mcg. The DV of zinc is 8 mg, and you could try up to 30 mg a day.

Herbs. A common symptom of hypothyroidism is low energy, and numerous Chinese herbs or herbal formulas may help you experience more vitality, perhaps through pathways that, at least in part, affect your thyroid. You'll get the most individualized herbal treatment from seeing an acupuncturist, but you could also try some formulas on your own. We've already mentioned one widely used formula for tonifying the qi, bu zhong yi qi tang. Other formulas aimed at boosting your qi are su jun zi tang and ba zhen tang.

Natural hormones and conventional medicine. Thyroid hormone is available only by prescription, either in the form of a natural extract of the thyroid gland of cows (bovine) or pigs (porcine), or as a synthetic product (i.e., levothyroxine); some professionals consider thyroid extract to be more effectively used by the body. If your thyroid is low, supplementing it can feel like a not-so-minor miracle, and a variety of ailments can disappear over a few months. At the same time, you should reduce or eliminate any other supplements directed at boosting thyroid, particularly tyrosine, so that the results of the hormone trial will be clear. While alternative means of supporting thyroid may be helpful, Jan generally recommends supplementing with pharmaceutical thyroid if testing has shown you are lacking this hormone. Whatever method(s) you choose in the spectrum of care, make sure you follow up with further testing to see if they are working.

Balancing Your Adrenal Hormones

The adrenals, two little walnut-shaped glands that sit on top of your kidneys, release hormones—notably cortisol, epinephrine, and norepinephrine*—that play key roles in guiding your body's responses to stress. With an acute stressor—let's say you're at the park with your preschooler, and she trips, scrapes her knee, and starts crying loudly—the hypothalamus tells the pituitary gland to signal the adrenals to send epinephrine and norepinephrine into your bloodstream, soon followed by cortisol. Ideally, when the stress is over—your daughter's recovered and playing happily again—both your knowledge that she's OK and the rising flood of stress hormones signal your hypothalamus and pituitary to tell the adrenals to settle back down. But with chronic stress, three problems can occur:†

- Your hypothalamus and pituitary could become so used to high levels of stress hormones that it takes increasing amounts to get these glands to stop ordering the adrenals to release more cortisol, etc. As a result, your mind may know that everything is alright—you see your daughter laughing happily in the sandbox—but your hypothalamus and pituitary glands, and thus your adrenals, aren't getting the message. Consequently, increasingly high levels of stress hormones could become the status quo in your body, even when no actual stressors are present: Now you feel routinely frazzled and "stressed out."
- The normal rhythm in your cortisol—low during the night so you can sleep, and higher in the morning to help you be active in the day—could become disturbed, making cortisol

---

* Epinephrine is another term for adrenaline, and norepinephrine is noradrenaline.

† These are simplified summaries of extremely complex processes that involve other aspects of the body as well, such as the hippocampus (a part of your brain).

peak around 4 a.m. and drop by lunchtime: Now you've got insomnia, and no pep at all in the afternoon.

- Your adrenal glands could become desensitized or "exhausted," so that they produce insufficient hormones even when the alarm bells are ringing: Now it feels harder than ever to kick into gear, and you may be more prone to allergies and joint pain (since cortisol inhibits inflammation). This state is sometimes termed *adrenal burnout* or *adrenal fatigue*, though these are not recognized medical diagnoses.

If you are experiencing any of these conditions, we suggest you do a relatively inexpensive, 24-hour salivary test of your cortisol and DHEA; your doctor or an endocrinologist can advise you about whether it makes sense to do additional, specialized assessments. Based on these findings, you could try one or more of the options in the spectrum of care that follows; many of them will not be specific to the three conditions above but will have a balancing effect in general. Meanwhile, try to reduce your stresses as best you can. Otherwise, any intervention will be like trying to fill a bucket with a hole in the bottom. Also take a look through the spectrum of care applied to other conditions for any suggestions that have a generally relaxing, destressing effect, such as exercise or 5-HTP. And try to get as much sleep as possible; even one night of poor sleep leads to elevated cortisol levels the next day.

Energetic. Studies have found that acupuncture can affect the hypothalamic-pituitary-adrenal (HPA) axis, often lowering the levels of circulating cortisol and other stress hormones.

Musculoskeletal. Yoga is a well-researched and powerful method of stress relief that can have a specific impact on the adrenal hormones. If you can arrange it, a good time for yoga is in the late afternoon or when you get home from work: It helps release the stress from your day and move you into a relaxed mindset for the evening. Sometimes children like to get in the act as well—at least for a few minutes—giving them some relaxation of their own.

Dietary. We tend to self-medicate when we're under stress—using caffeine, alcohol, or recreational drugs. Besides the long-term problems this causes, it can mask a growing disturbance in the HPA axis. Try eliminating caffeine, alcohol, or other drugs for a few days and see how you do; the results could be a wake-up call that you need to make a more serious effort to manage your stresses or tend to your adrenals. At a minimum, try not to exceed a couple cups of coffee and/or one drink of alcohol per day.

One potential source of cortisol rising at night and waking you up is blood sugar slumping then—which stimulates cortisol secretion—if it has been surging during the day. To reduce those surges, try eliminating or radically reducing sugar and refined carbohydrates for a week while eating more protein, and see if that helps.

Supplements. A deficiency of pantothenic acid—vitamin B5—can weaken the adrenal glands, and the IDD of 500–1,000 mg could help them increase cortisol production. Chronic stress depletes vitamin C, and this vitamin (as well as the B-vitamins) supports adrenal function. The IDD for vitamin C is to start with 2,000 mg in divided doses and increase slowly up to bowel tolerance (the amount just below that which causes diarrhea).

The amino acid tyrosine is the precursor to norepinephrine (as well as dopamine), and studies have shown it to improve the adaptation to stress. A reasonable daily dose would be to start with 500 mg taken before noon, and increase slowly to about 1 gram. On the other hand, Jan has observed that women who tend to be sensitive or nervous often don't like tyrosine—they find it too stimulating. So, always check in with yourself, and don't push something that doesn't feel right.

Another nutrient that could help balance the stress feedback system in your body is phosphatidylserine (PS), in doses of 100–200 mg per day.*

If stress has thrown off your sleep clock, you could try methylcobalamin, the active coenzyme form of vitamin B12. It is particularly effective when used in combination with 20 minutes or more of bright light between 6 and 8 a.m. See if you can get out for a brief walk at that time—which will be relaxing in its own right!

Herbs. Panax and Siberian ginseng appear to have an adaptogenic effect on the adrenal glands, both lifting low levels and decreasing high levels. Unfortunately, the dosage required for this function is poorly researched in humans, in part because the potency of ginseng varies greatly depending on the source and the preparation. We suggest starting with 500 mg/day of dried herb from a reputable company and perhaps increasing slowly up to 2,000–3,000 mg/day. It's generally best not to take ginseng in the evening, to avoid an overly stimulating result.

Licorice binds to the hormone receptors of cortisol, creating a cortisol-like effect. You could initially try 100–300 mg/day, and perhaps increase slowly to 1,000 mg. In about a fifth of the population, high doses of licorice lead to hypertension, so you should take this herb under the supervision of a licensed health care provider, and check your blood pressure frequently when you first start using it.

Natural hormones and conventional medicine. To restore a normal sleep cycle, you could use melatonin, 0.5–1 mg taken orally or sublingually 30 to 60 minutes before bedtime, and some practitioners may recommend taking higher doses. In cases of severe adrenal fatigue, hydrocortisone can be given in dosages that approximate the body's normal production of cortisol. If you need it, this treatment can feel

* Some studies used 800 mg, but we have no experience with that dosage.

beneficial, but it should be initiated only by a doctor who is familiar with it.

YOUR IMMUNE SYSTEM

Day and night, the immune system works to keep bacteria, viruses, parasites, and toxic chemicals from invading your body and causing disease, as well as destroy abnormal cells that might become cancerous. It is the primary defender of your health, and it has two arms:*

- **Innate:** This includes your body's soft armor (the skin and mucus membranes), large cells (such as macrophages) that engulf microorganisms and toxins, and chemicals that kill or disable microbes.
- **Adaptive:** This part of your immune system "learns" to recognize and attack microbes, diseased cells, or foreign substances, sometimes using parts of the innate immune system to assist it. Its elements include:
    - — Antibodies: molecules that mark an antigen (the molecular fingerprint of a microorganism, cell, or chemical) and guide an attack
    - — B-cells: white blood cells that produce antibodies
    - — T-cells: three types of white blood cells that kill diseased cells, or activate or inhibit other parts of the immune system
    - — Thymus gland: transforms immature T-cells into mature ones that can tell the difference between "self" and "nonself," and secretes hormones that help guide the immune system

---

* This description of the immune system is simplified, focusing mainly on those elements that will be discussed further.

When your immune system goes into action, the results can include inflammation (enabling your defenders to get to the battlefield), mucus production, fever (which helps kill heat-sensitive microbes), and fatigue (so you'll rest and your body can heal). But they could also include misguided assaults on neutral substances (allergies) or the body's own tissues (autoimmune disease).

What Can Disturb the Immune System

The key to a healthy immune system is balance, so that it is vigilant and powerful yet also discerning and controlled. Let's see how bearing and rearing children can wear down and disturb your immune system, making it like a weary soldier lurching into battle, too depleted to defend herself and too rattled to distinguish friend from foe.

Stress. Your stresses make your immune system both weaker and more prone to overreact. First, stress stimulates the release of corticosteroid hormones, and these suppress both arms of your immune system so it's less able to ward off invading viruses, bacteria, or parasites. Second, a woman's immune system is generally more active than a man's is, so it's easier for stress to make it overreactive. For example, stress increases the release of histamines within your body, causing inflammation signals to be sent out as a shout instead of a whisper. As a result, an allergen that would once give you no more than a few sneezes could now lead to hives or asthma. Stress also seems to play a role in the development and severity of autoimmune illnesses, which are more likely in women after they have children.

Nutritional deficits. Like an army at war, your immune system consumes resources at an amazing rate when it fights an infection. For example, an activated B-cell can produce about a thousand antibody molecules per second before dying in a day or two. Therefore, the immune system needs a big stockpile of nutrients. But if your body has become depleted, a lack of protein or a deficit in any one of numerous nutrients—such as vitamin C, vitamin D, or zinc—will lower its resistance to disease.

Fetal tissue. Long after you've given birth, some cells from your baby will normally remain within your body. It is possible that the immune system may interpret those fetal cells as "foreign," putting it on red alert, now more likely to overreact and develop an autoimmune disease.

Other systems of the body. Disturbed digestion can decrease the absorption of the vital nutrients your immune system needs. Additionally, GI disturbance increases the chance of developing food sensitivities, which activate your immune system needlessly.

Similarly, changes in the nervous system due to motherhood can reduce the potency of your immune responses. Depression, for instance, is associated with a slower rate of recovery from illness and less effective white blood cell activity.

Hormones bind to immune cells throughout your body, sometimes telling them to hit the gas and other times the brakes. For example, low estrogen can reduce the effectiveness of your immune system. On the other hand, healthy levels of estrogen, progesterone, oxytocin, and prolactin help control overzealous immune function. Rapid fluctuations in these hormones—from stress, weaning, new pregnancies, etc.—can lead to hair-trigger immune responses, increasing the chance of an autoimmune disease.

Signs and Symptoms of Disturbance in the Immune System

Fundamentally, depletion can weaken your immune system—reducing its response to infection—and disturb it, so it is more likely to attack innocent bystanders (allergies) or your own tissues (autoimmune reactions).

Reduced response. If your immune system is weakened, you would be more prone to frequent, severe, and lingering diseases, from the common cold to serious infections.

Allergic reactions. As we've seen, an overly reactive immune system can intensify your body's response to allergens.

Autoimmune disease. When the body is attacked by its own immune system, the general symptoms typically include fatigue and inflammation. The specific symptoms vary, depending on the illness.

Assessment of the Immune System

Routine office visits with your doctor do not usually detect subtle abnormalities in the status of your immune system. These are diagnosed with tests that doctors generally order only if you mention some of the signs and symptoms described previously. Basic tests of immune function include a complete blood count (CBC), white blood cell count (WBC), C-reactive protein (CRP), and sedimentation rate (a general index of inflammation). Additional tests can assess specialized elements of the immune system, such as helper T-cells. And on your own, you can investigate any food sensitivities as we've previously discussed.

Strengthening and Balancing Your Immune System

Probably the single most important thing you can do for your immune system is mental, not physical: A positive outlook, social support, and low stress will nurture the healing powers of your body. Since angry quarrels depress immune system function, you'll also benefit from finding positive ways to work out issues with your partner (covered in the next three chapters). Second, promoting your overall wellness will support your immune system in numerous ways. In particular, try to get lots of deep sleep, since that's when your brain and body produce several substances that enhance immune function. Good nutrition and a balanced digestive tract are also vital allies to a potent immune system. Third, you'll want to keep the overall load on your immune system as low as possible by minimizing your exposure to toxins, allergens (including foods to which you are sensitive), or infection so that it is not already burdened when new challenges come along.

On this foundation, let's look at the options within the spectrum of care for strengthening and balancing your immune system. Some of these are preventive, while others help the immune system when it is being attacked or disturbed.

Energetic. Acupuncture can help restore and maintain a healthy homeostasis in the immune system.

Musculoskeletal. Moderate exercise boosts the levels of several kinds of white blood cells, but strenuous exercise—like running a 10K race—briefly reduces lymphocytes, natural killer cells, and antibodies in your respiratory and digestive tracts. If you're interested in something a little more relaxed, massage and even affectionate touching have also been shown to increase immune system function.

Dietary. You really can turbocharge your immune system with every bite you eat. Lots of vegetables and a reasonable amount of fruit will give you immune-boosting carotenoids and flavonoids. A solid serving of protein at every meal will also help keep your immune system humming along. And it's critical to minimize sugar and refined flours. Besides wearing on your body in general and thus affecting the immune system indirectly, sugars have direct effects as well. For instance, studies found that consuming about two sodas' worth of sugar knocked down the effectiveness of white blood cells by roughly 50 percent within 1 hour, with residual effects lasting for several more hours. Finally, a low-fat diet with minimal caffeine has also been shown to improve immune function.

Supplements. The immune system requires a full cupboard of nutrients in your body, so we'll repeat our recommendation that you take a high potency multivitamin/mineral supplement every day. Depending on what your supplement contains, you may want to add one or more of the following nutrients.

- **Antioxidants:** These nutrients aid your immune system in numerous ways. They are generally most effective in combination with one another, but you can also use them individually:
  - *Vitamin A* plays an essential role in nourishing the skin and mucus membranes, your primary barriers against infection; the micellized form is easily absorbable. It also stimulates white blood cell activity and antibody response. Do not exceed the MSDV, and do not supplement vitamin A if you are or might become pregnant.
  - *Vitamin C* supports many aspects of the immune system, including white blood cells, interferon, and secretion of thymic hormones. For maximum immune support, you could try the IDD, taking increasing quantities of vitamin C up to the point that you develop diarrhea, and then lower the dose until normal bowel function is restored.
  - *Vitamin E* (primarily taken as gamma-tocopherol) seems to help both antibody-related and cell-mediated aspects of the immune system. You could increase the MSDV to the IDD of 800 IU.
  - *Carotenoids* are best consumed through eating 5–7 servings of vegetables each day. If you use supplements, take a product with mixed carotenoids, since high doses of beta-carotene alone may, in some cases, be harmful.
  - *Quercetin* is useful for settling the immune system and reducing the symptoms of allergies and food sensitivities;

try 400–500 mg, 1–3 times a day, ideally taken before meals.

- **B-vitamins:** A deficiency in nearly any B-vitamin will weaken the immune system, and vitamin B6, vitamin B12, and folic acid are particularly important. The levels of the B-vitamins in the MSDV will support proper immune function. For an extra boost, you could increase them up to the IDD we've previously discussed.
- **Vitamin D:** This helps activate immune defenses such as T cells while also regulating inflammation and preventing autoimmune activations. Start with the MSDV while also getting your vitamin D levels tested; Jan has found that some people need to go up to the IDDs for a while in order to develop appropriate levels of this vitamin.
- **Minerals:** Several minerals have a striking ability to support your immune system:
  — *Iron deficiency* (even when minimal) lessens the effectiveness of several parts of your immune system. Unfortunately, low iron levels are widespread among women in general, and mothers in particular can have a shortage of iron due to the lingering effects of pregnancy. Getting more iron into your body is best accomplished through eating liver; since toxins concentrate in the liver, try to get this meat from beef or chickens raised on organic foods and no artificial chemicals. The next best source of iron is a chelated supplement, such as iron bisglycinate. If you are already taking the MSDV of iron and testing shows that your body is still deficient, you could take an IDD of 30 mg twice a day. But don't take more than the MSDVs of iron unless your body is clearly lacking in this mineral, since high amounts of iron can be toxic.

- *Selenium shortages* weaken many aspects of the immune system. Even when blood levels of selenium are normal, taking 200 mcg per day has been shown to help the immune response.
- *Zinc deficiency* has been found to decrease immune system activity, while supplementation has been shown to enhance it. For purposes of preventing illness, you could take 30 mg of zinc citrate, picolinate, or gluconate. If you feel a cold coming on, zinc lozenges can be helpful (about 25 mg every 2 hours up to about 250 mg per day); one study found this dosing shortened the duration of colds by 64 percent. But do this for only a few days.

Herbs. Astragalus is used in Chinese medicine as a long-term immune tonic and for active viral infections, and you can usually buy it in a health food store; for dosing, follow the instructions on the package. Echinacea has been shown to boost the immune system, particularly when used at the beginning of a cold, flu, or respiratory infection. It should be taken in small doses, about ⅛ teaspoon of a 1:5 tincture, every few hours, for at most 6 weeks. Do not use this herb if you are prone to allergies or have an autoimmune disease since it might overstimulate your immune system.

Probiotics. By helping balance the microbial ecology of your GI system, probiotics can support your immune system indirectly. Additionally, there are intriguing indications that certain probiotics, such as lactobacillus, can stimulate the innate immune system, making it more active in fighting off invading microbes. For suggestions about taking probiotics please see pages 203–204.

✧ ✧ ✧

Motherhood is startling in its sheer physicality, from the first swelling in your belly to the crick in your neck while holding your baby perfectly still so she won't wake up again, and to the long-term depletion many women experience after having children. Those oh-so-tangible effects can take you by surprise and make you feel vulnerable. They're humbling, and they fly in the face of the perfectionistic expectations many women have for themselves.

Everyone has frailties, yet sometimes it's hard to acknowledge your own to others, or even within your own heart. But that's what's needed for compassion—for yourself, and for your body: Your mind and your body are both hardworking, weary, and deserving of loving care. A clear-eyed respect for your body's needs can help you feel that it's right to ask for and receive support from others for any health problems. In the next three chapters, we'll explore how to cultivate a supportive, loving relationship with your partner—for its own sake, and as an important resource for your lasting health.

PART FOUR

Nurturing Your Intimate Relationship

A marriage has two fundamental aspects—a practical partnership and an intimate friendship—and children can't help but challenge each of them.

Regarding the first of these, kids bring hard questions that good-hearted and otherwise like-minded partners often disagree about, from the best way to help a baby sleep through the night to how to pay for college. The total workload jumps dramatically, yet you probably can't call on a village of "helper moms" that would have supported your family in past generations. Much of what once would have been carried by many has now shifted to one, your partner, but if he doesn't shoulder that burden, it all falls onto you.

In the intimate parts of your relationship, after children arrive it's understandably harder to find time or energy for fun together, good conversation, or sweet lovemaking. Issues from the practical partnership—such as arguments over how to parent the kids or divide the workload fairly—impact any intimate friendship. And issues from it—whether it's the depth of conversation or the frequency of sex—spill over onto the practical partnership, adding heat and smoke to subjects that are often already challenging.

As a result, even with the best of intentions, it is common for a mother and father to have conflicts about some matter of child-rearing or sharing the load, and to experience a loss of intimacy. Besides being upsetting, all this can wear on your health. For example, quarrels increase blood pressure, wear down the immune system, and disturb a person's hormones. The way spouses treat each other when the children are little will shape their relationship for many years, and in the extreme, it can tear a marriage apart. If the couple stays together, an atmosphere of tension and emotional distance increases the risk that their children will feel insecure and develop psychological problems.

Therefore, it is vital for parents to be strong partners, and the next three chapters are designed to give you the tools you need to keep your relationship moving in a good direction or to get it back on track it if it has gotten derailed. Chapter 6 covers skillful communication, chapter 7 addresses the practical partnership, and chapter 8 focuses on the intimate friendship. Ideally, your partner will read these. (If you are living apart from the father of your children, or with another person who is helping raise your kids, you can adapt them to your situation.) But we know that this may not happen, so we wrote them to be used either together or by you alone. Used by just you, they will help you see more clearly what you have a right to ask for and how to do so more effectively. And you can learn how to be a more skillful partner yourself in order to draw out the best in him, address his concerns and needs, and know that you have done the best you could in your relationship.

Of course, it may feel doubly burdensome to have to learn new skills in order to get your partner to do what you think he should have done in the first place. But the alternative is to feel immobilized and resentful while matters stay the same or get worse. If you make an effort, things are likely to improve. It will help you feel better to be active, rather than passive, in your relationship, and it is better for your children to see you sticking up for yourself. Even in the saddest scenario—if your marriage was already in the intensive care unit and nothing could revive it—the skills you will learn by trying will help you with both your ex-husband and any future partners.

But it's much more likely that your efforts will help increase or bring back the good feelings you and your partner have had for each other. Over and over, we've seen that just a few small changes—a little more understanding, a little more skill in communicating, a little more support—can make a huge difference in a relationship.

CHAPTER SIX

Talking with Your Partner

It is an amazing but true thing that practically the only people who ever say mean, insulting, wounding things to us are those of our own households.

Dorothea Dix

Sometimes talking about the simplest thing is like walking through a minefield. For example, imagine a father coming home from work to his wife who has been alone with their young child much of the day, and they've grown so irritated with each other that this dialogue is pretty typical:

He: [walks through the door, sees some clutter, and mutters to himself] *What a mess.*

She: [stung by the criticism after having spent many hours alone with their daughter] *There you go, always criticizing when you first get home.*

He: *You're so messy it drives me crazy.*

She: *I don't see* you *lifting a finger to help.*

He: [walks over and puts a toy on a shelf] *There, I helped. Now are you happy?*

She: [under her breath] *Such a jerk.*

He: *Well, there you go again, losing control. You can't talk without getting hysterical.*

She: *Your mother spoiled you rotten, but I don't have to take your crap.*

He: [yelling] *Once and for all, stop talking about my family. Or I've had it!*

A CIVIL TONGUE

Thirty years of research have shown that the key to a loving and lasting relationship is how the two people interact with each other. Positive exchanges build up an emotional bank account of trust and warmth, and they make it easier to get through a conflict without anyone losing their temper. In strong couples, positive interactions really outnumber the negative ones.

An interaction is like a rally in tennis, and civility is what keeps the ball in bounds. Each time it is your turn to "hit the ball," you have choices about how you hear what was said and how you respond. First, in terms of how you receive what comes over the "net," you could focus on the most useful or accurate parts of their communication. This would help you see the best in the other person and feel more hopeful and calm. Or you could fixate on the parts that are exaggerated, inaccurate, or inflammatory, which would increase your sense of being misunderstood, attacked, hurt, or angry. Second, in terms of how you respond, you could send back the most constructive communication possible—given what came at you—which would preserve your dignity, put you in a good light, and give your partner something positive to work with. Or you could fire back with some nasty topspin, losing your cool, clouding the issues, and motivating the other person to retaliate in kind. In sum, each of you could build on the positive, or go negative on the negative.

Besides feeling awful, negative interactions stress your body and deplete you further. An atmosphere of conflict between their parents worries children, and it's a risk factor for them developing depression, anxiety, and behavior problems. Frequent quarrels also wear down marital bonds. Every ugly, nasty little exchange makes each person more sensitive to the next one, the same way repeated chafing of the skin makes it increasingly tender to the touch, so even a light bump feels harshly abrasive. Then partners can trigger each other in runaway chain reactions. On the other hand, civility interrupts the cycle of negativity, even if just one person does it.

Disagreements are natural in any relationship, and they usually increase after children. Civility does not prevent you from speaking your mind. It just helps you make your point better and increases the chance that you'll actually be heard.

How to Make a Conversation Go Badly

Let's look first at what went wrong in the interaction that opened this chapter, and then at how it could have gone better.

- **Leading with the negative, making no emotional connection** (*What a mess!*): If the first statement is negative, the other person will feel jolted and attacked. There also needs to be some stage-setting that makes an emotional connection and finds out if this is a good time to talk.

- **Overstatement** (*There you go, always criticizing when you first get home.*): The speaker makes it sound like *you do this entirely bad thing all the time in every way* when she uses words like *always* or *never,* and when she does not use qualifying, softening language such as *often, around bedtimes,* or *when you're watching TV.*
- **Blaming** (*You're so messy it drives me crazy.*): A fault-finding attack is shaming and hurtful, and usually triggers an angry defense.
- **Counterattack** (*I don't see* you *lifting a finger to help.*): This both escalates the conflict and introduces a new topic. When multiple topics swirl around in a murky soup, nothing gets accomplished.
- ***Reductio ad absurdum*** (*There, I helped. Now are you happy?*): "Reducing to absurdity" deflates others by making their wish, complaint, or idea sound foolish. That's hurtful in itself, plus it's only a short and explosive step from *your view is ridiculous* to *YOU are ridiculous.*
- **Insults** (*Such a jerk.*): Long after an argument is over, insults linger in the mind like emotional napalm, part glue and part gasoline, sticking and burning. Frequent insults are emotional abuse, a grinding assault on the other person's sense of worth.
- **Character attacks** (*Well, there you go again, losing control. You can't talk without getting hysterical.*): There's a world of difference between saying *What you did was bad* and *YOU are bad.* When one person takes shots at the overall character of another, the target of the attack feels that his or her good parts are overlooked or even negated, and is likely to fire back in kind.
- **Side issues** (*Your mother spoiled you rotten, but I don't have to take your crap.*): These are distractions that shift the focus away from the real issue.

- **Demands** (*Once and for all, stop talking about my family!*): Every communication contains two messages: the explicit content and an implicit statement about the relationship between the speaker and listener. We all have deep needs to feel both autonomous and connected in our relationships. When the implicit message threatens either need, that becomes the overriding issue. For example, any demand says implicitly, *I get to boss you around and limit your autonomy.* Most people fight back against attempts at dominance, which turns up the heat and diverts attention from the explicit topic.
- **Threats** (*Or I've had it!*): Both the explicit meaning of a threat, that something bad could happen, and the implicit one that *I get to intimidate you* are alarming. Threats crowd out other issues and foster threats in return, such as: *Fine! Just see what your relationship with the kids is like if you do!*

How to Help a Conversation Go Well

The key to a good conversation is each person's purpose. For example, is it your intention to speak your truth clearly, find out what is really bugging your partner, discover what you need to do differently, and solve problems? Or is it to avoid responsibility, dump your reactions on the other person, look good, or win? In your heart, where do you truly want to be coming from?

When each person's intentions are positive, they find ways to connect and mend, rather than diverge and wound. A good conversation may start messy and heated, with a flurry of diverging volleys, but then one or both partners starts to settle down, and they converge on mutual understanding and practical solutions. Let's replay the dialogue above, but this time with each partner keeping a civil tongue:

- **Start by connecting.**

He: [Walks through the front door. Sees the mess, feels like grumbling, but thinks better of it. Takes a big breath. Picks up his daughter and jiggles her in his arms while she giggles and makes him laugh. Smiles at his wife.] *How'd it go?* [They chat for a few minutes. He says something nice about what she did that day. There's a pause, and he takes the plunge.] *I don't want to hassle you, but could we talk about the clutter?*

Leading with connection sends the reassuring, implicit message that *we are together, you matter to me.* Whenever you can, start by joining with your partner, rather than detaching or distancing, through warmth, touch, showing interest or concern, or saying what you agree with from the outset. And see if you can keep that sense of connection going.

- **Speak with accuracy and restraint.**

She: [Warily, but with a touch of humor.] *You're doing pretty well—this is the first time you've complained about that this week.*

You can usually take your time to think before you speak and avoid exaggerated or inflammatory language. You can explain how intensely you feel or how important something is to you by scaling it, as in: *On a 10-point scale of bothering me, this is just a 3.* Imagining that the conversation is videotaped could help you avoid saying something that would make you wince later.

- **Take responsibility.**

He: [Knows the subject is charged, so he takes the time to say clearly how he feels.] *I know Caitlin's a little mess machine and you're doing the best you can. It's just that things are chaotic at work and the commute's more stressful than ever, so I'm hoping for orderliness at home. Plus we've already talked about you picking up before I get home. When it's still a mess, it feels like what I say doesn't matter.*

When you talk about your own experience, using mainly "I statements," your partner will understand you better and will be less likely to feel attacked. People can argue with your opinions or plans, but your experience is *your* experience; it has an inherent validity that does not need to be justified or defended.

- **Stay on topic.**

She: [Starts feeling defensive and wanting to shift the topic to how Caitlin was especially active that day but catches herself.] *OK. Let's talk about this. I also want to think with you about starting Caitlin in preschool. Can we talk about that later tonight? She's getting so restless at home. I put one toy away and meanwhile she's taken out two others.*

Try to finish one issue before moving on to another. Sometimes it helps to set a time limit: *Let's do 10 minutes on how I need to get the house straighter by the time you get here, and then 10 minutes on how you need to come home on time.*

- **Focus on what is accurate or useful in what the other person is saying.**

He: [Thinks she's trying to justify herself by talking about Caitlin and starts to veer off topic to rebut that point, but he knows that would just get them fighting, so he stops himself.] *You're right, Caitlin is getting real active. I know that makes it harder to straighten up, so let's talk about preschool later. But you have to admit, when you're firm with her, she behaves better.*

When you can, begin your response with what you like or agree with about what the other person has said. Emphasizing common ground conveys respect and moves you toward positive solutions.

- **Keep your dignity.**

  She: [Liked the first part of what he said, but then he slipped in that last bit about being firmer with their daughter. Feels her heart start to pound. Speaks with intensity but maintains self-control.] *Look, I really don't like hearing about how I ought to be firmer with Caitlin. You try spending day after day with a two-year-old. You don't do that—no criticism, just fact—so you have* no idea *what it's like. You just can't be firm every second. Please don't be so free with your advice. I am actually quite firm with Caitlin, and you know that people say she's well behaved.*

  You could recall someone who embodies an attitude of self-respect and uprightness in the face of provocation and imagine speaking in the same manner. You can talk in a way that makes you feel proud of yourself.

- **Address concrete specifics.**

  He: [Resists the temptation to re-fight old quarrels, and he refocuses the conversation.] *OK, OK. I know you're pretty firm, though I wish you were 10 percent firmer. But that's not the issue. Here's my basic point: I don't really care about the rest of the house. I'd just like to be able to walk through the front door into a living room that is peaceful and orderly. And I thought we'd agreed you'd straighten that up before I got home.*

  Nothing can be done about a vague complaint or a broad assault on someone's character. But you *can* solve well-defined problems. For example, you can clarify how much of a change you want, as the father did above with his "10 percent" comment.

- **Concede points when you can.**

  She: [Still calming down from the "you're not firm enough" side-issue. Considers arguing with whether she needs to be "10 percent firmer," but thinks better of it.] *You're right, I did say I'd keep things cleaner. I didn't realize you only care about the living room. That's doable. But I have to tell you, I want more respect for how I am raising Caitlin, with more understanding for what it's like to be home alone with her much of the day.*

If it is more important to you to discover what is true and what will work than it is to be right or to win a power struggle, you can be good-humored about conceding a point. Plus that's the fastest way to get the other person to stop pressing their point. The true winner of an argument is the one who learns the most.

✦ **Make requests, not demands, and agreements, not threats.**

He: [Wants to fire back but has learned that the impulse to do so is actually an internal big, flashing warning to buy some time until he has calmed down.] *Hmm. Let me think about that for a minute.* [Discreetly takes a few big breaths. Thinks about whether he's gone overboard. Remembers that people do say that Caitlin is well behaved for a two-year-old. Remembers the time he had Caitlin for most of a Saturday and how he had to loosen up on the rules. Looks at his wife and feels compassion for her, pulled in one direction by their daughter and in another direction by him.] *OK. Would this work: Picked-up living room, so-so rest of house, and we try your firmness level for a while?*

She: [Still irritated. But softened by his tone and partial giving in. Considers whether she can actually get the living room straightened up by the time he gets home, and makes a counterproposal.] *Well, I like where you're going. But what if you're late and Caitlin leaves out some new stuff, and you yell at me about it?*

He: [Sees her basic point and doesn't get distracted by the exaggeration about yelling. Nods and smiles.] *You're right, that wouldn't be good.*

She: *I can keep it picked up between 6:00 and 6:30. If you get home later, all bets are off. OK?*

He: *Sounds like a plan. I'm tired of arguing, anyway!*

How to Be Civil

Lead with the positive.

Make a connection.

Speak with accuracy and restraint.

Take personal responsibility. Lean toward the 80-20 rule: Focus 80 percent on yourself and 20 percent on your partner.

Stay on topic.

Don't interrupt.

Focus on what is true and useful.

Keep your dignity.

Address concrete specifics.

Concede points when you can.

Make requests, not demands.

Make agreements, not threats.

If People Are Getting Upset

It's hard to be civil when the need is greatest: when reactions are getting intense. But you can help yourself in many ways. You might like to take a quick look back at the methods for coping with upsetting experiences in chapters 2 and 3. The following suggestions build on that foundation to focus on your relationship, and each one is also something you can ask for from your partner.

Stepping back. When you step back from your reactions, that is the beginning of *you* being in control, not them. See if you can observe your body sensations, wants, emotions, and thoughts. Rather than *being* your reactions—identified with them and hijacked by them—you can *have* them, with some space around them and distance from them. A simple powerful way to do this is to name them softly to yourself, such as: *irritated . . . hurt . . . scared . . . want to get away . . . wish he wouldn't talk to me that way. . . .* With practice, you will get better and better at it—and raising a family will give you plenty of practice!

You can step back from the other person's reactions, too. You could remind yourself that you are separate, perhaps imagining a boundary between you like a picket fence or, if need be, a thick wall. Or visualize a shield around you, like one of those force fields in science fiction, that blocks anything negative; you have total control over this shield and only you decide what gets through. You could imagine that you are looking at other people through the wrong end of a telescope, so they seem small and far away, or that you are turning the volume knob down on their voices. You can let their words or feelings move through you like wind ruffling the leaves on a tree; when the breeze has passed, you are still here and can decide for yourself what is accurate or useful in what they've said. Perhaps lighten up the seriousness or intensity by visualizing them wearing funny hats. You could also look past the most provocative words to the softer feelings and wants that lie beneath, using the empathy skills discussed in the next section.

When it's your turn to talk, you know your partner's hot buttons, and you can usually make your point without punching them. Clarify from the outset that you are not blaming or criticizing him (unless you truly intend to). Be careful how the issue is being framed, which is often what irritates most, and put it back in the proper context if necessary. For instance, are you approaching him as a normally on-top-of-it dad who slipped up, or as a perennial klutz? You can anticipate his concerns: *I'm not suggesting we take Steve out of soccer. I'm just wondering if there is a way for him not to get so banged up when he plays.* Try to be aware of the presence of implicit negative messages such as *I know more than you, you blew it,* or *I'm the boss here.* Remember that he, like you, has worries or doubts that can be reassured with messages such as *I've really appreciated how good you are with the baby* or *I know you've been working hard to make more money.*

Working with your body. The stress relief techniques in chapter 2 can help calm down your body, such as breathing from the diaphragm, tensing and then relaxing, or imagining the upset draining out like liquid through valves at the ends of your fingers and toes. Sometimes a person's body is so upset that there is no sense in even talking. Come back to the issue later, maybe after you've taken a walk around the block.

Working with your emotions. Of all the emotions, anger is usually the most challenging for a couple. On the one hand, suppressing it feels bad, plus it denies the other person important information. On the other hand, anger crowds out other messages, makes partners back away from each other, and breeds anger in turn. As an experiment, you—and hopefully he, as well—could try not to speak in an angry way for a day or two, or even longer, and see what happens to the atmosphere in your home. You can still explain what's bothering you, but you'll find yourself pausing longer before you speak and talking in a more heartfelt way. (Over the long run, of course, you will have to make some headway with the specific situations that are frustrating and irritating; this is covered in the next two chapters.)

Working with the mind. Our experiences growing up can't help but color our relationships. For example, people who were criticized a lot or even verbally abused as children are likely to have old feelings of hurt and anger well up in an argument with their mate. You can use the questions in the box to help sort your reactions into those that are proportionate to what is actually happening here and now, and into those that are transferred into the current situation from childhood (for more examples of this method, see chapters 2 and 3). Then, when it gets intense, you will be more able to help yourself and your partner by saying something like: *Look, part of my reaction here comes from getting yelled at as a kid, but still, I don't think you should use that tone of voice with me, especially about something as minor as dirty dishes.*

How Childhood Affects Reactions to a Partner

Consider the questions below for yourself. Then, if you like, you could apply them to your partner.

Your feelings as a child: *What did your parents do that hurt, angered, or otherwise upset you? How do these emotional reactions to your parents come up when your partner acts similarly?*

Your wants as a child: *How did you feel about how your parents responded to your wants as a child? How do those reactions come into play today when your partner responds to your wants? What did you yearn for that you long for today from your partner?*

Seeing your parents together: *How did your mother act toward your father, especially when things were tense? Do you react to your partner in any similar ways? How did your father act toward your mother? How do you react today if your partner treats you in similar ways?*

This idea of sorting is useful in other ways as well. Try to zero in on the current issue in its own right, not linked to other situations that make it seem like everything's all falling apart. For example, a mother told Jan this story: *On the way home one night, Antonio forgot to buy a special jar of baby food, and I got really mad. He was apologetic and ready to zip out to the market, but all I could do was think about other times when his mind was clearly elsewhere. What was really just a half-hour delay in getting a jar of baby food became a huge issue.*

You can also separate out the ways that your reactions have been shaded or amplified by your temperament. Let's say you have an anxious disposition, and today your husband says, *Tommy needs a bigger bike.* You could notice how your underlying temperament shifts your response toward excessive alarm. These are perfectly normal reactions. But for yourself and your partner, try to keep in mind the true scale of the problem: *I'm getting worried about this, even though I know we can afford it, especially if we can pick up a used bike at a yard sale. I get so anxious about money. But I guess we can figure this out.*

Sorting things out. You can sort out where your partner has a role in the topic of your conversation from where he does not, by saying something like: *Our overall situation is tough, but nobody's the bad guy. The only part that is about you in what I'm saying is that it would really help if you could pick up Sophie at day care.* You'll be anticipating the questions any listener might have: *What does this have to do with* me*? Is there something I need to do? Are you saying I screwed up?* Make it clear whether you want him to simply listen, or to help you solve a problem outside the family (e.g., with work or a relative), or to change the way he's been acting.

Then, sort out the specific ways he's involved by distinguishing *faults* from *putting in correction* or *gracious gifts*. A fault exists when a person falls short of a reasonable moral standard, such as not keeping an agreement with a partner or getting too angry with a child. Putting in correction means becoming more skillful in the future without being at fault about the past: no blame, but there's a better way. A gracious gift is when you do something nice for its own sake, not to remedy a fault or a lack of skill. Suppose your husband drives faster on the freeway than you are comfortable with. But let's also suppose that he's not reckless, and most other drivers are going as fast or faster. You could ask him to shave 5 miles an hour off his pace when you or the children are in the car as a favor that would make you feel less stressed, not because there is anything wrong about the way he drives.

No one likes being at fault, in the wrong, to blame, the bad guy, and so on. Since (hopefully) each partner cares more about things going better in the future than making the other person feel bad about the past, why not cut to the chase and go for what each of you wants without complicating things by trying to make the other person agree that he or she was, in fact, a jerk? For an example of how to do this, let's go back to Sophie and day care: *Look, I'm not saying you should feel horribly guilty when you're late getting Sophie* [making it clear there's no fault]. *But you've said it yourself that you want to improve at wrapping things up in time to get out of the office by 5:30* [putting in correction]. *Plus it will be really nice for Sophie and me to have more time together with you at home* [asking for a gracious gift].

If your partner thinks *you* are at fault and you do not agree, try to be active within your own mind, a free agent who can decide for herself what is true or not, what's his stuff and what's your own, how your own personal code applies to the situation, and what you are going to do differently—if at all—in the future. When we get defensive, treating the other person's communication like an unwanted message, they usually try harder to deliver it! Paradoxically, the fastest way to get someone's grievance to move on is first to let it move in:

- Really hear the complaint.
- Take the maximum reasonable personal responsibility for it.
- Express the maximum reasonable remorse or apology.
- Commit to appropriate changes from this point on.

This approach is *not* weak. Actually, it is a strong way to act in your self-interest.

Staying in bounds. It might help to agree on some basic ground rules for talking together, such as no name-calling, yelling, or threats.

You could agree in advance to take a break if one or both of you needs to calm down; the person who calls time-out should propose a specific time to speak again.

During a quarrel, follow the ground rules yourself, and if your partner does not, ask him to; if you can, speak from your heart about how you feel when he talks that way. If he continues to break the ground rules, you could call time-out, and if necessary, walk away. Fundamentally, all you can control is how *you* speak, and your civility will create the best chance that other people will communicate in more civil ways themselves.

A change of setting can foster civility, like going for a walk together or sitting in a coffee shop. A well-considered text or a voice message can get your thoughts in order and express them through a buffer that may make it easier for your partner to truly hear you. On the other hand, it's best to avoid texting or emailing in the heat of strong feelings, since tone and nuance are so easily misunderstood. It might help to propose recording a conversation, both to learn from later and because it puts people on their best behavior.

Having another person present while you discuss a touchy subject can be calming: perhaps a clergy member, trusted friend, or therapist, but not your children. A professional is especially called for if there is emotional abuse, drug or alcohol problems, frequent contempt or criticism, or intense fights in front of the children.

If there is actual or threatened violence—the ultimate breach of civility—you should immediately tell a physician, clergy member, therapist, or the police, or call a shelter. Shelters, including emergency housing for children and family safety programs, are listed online or accessible through 24-hour hotlines. Domestic abuse is, sadly, not uncommon: About one woman in three will be seriously assaulted at least once by her partner, and the odds of this increase—sadder still—if there are children in the home. It might feel shameful to admit that you're having to deal with this, but literally millions of other women have been in a similar situation. You're not alone, it's not your fault, and the most important thing of all is for you to tell someone who cares about you. It's usually wisest to start with support for you and then later on perhaps involve your partner (rather than the first step being couples therapy).

In less serious situations, consider agreeing on a "no-fight rule" for several weeks. Civil disagreements are alright, but if they escalate at all, you would both stop and regroup. This is an admittedly artificial and short-term arrangement, like a cast on a broken arm. It allows the stress chemistry in your bodies to settle down while you build up a recent history of at least neutral interactions. If you add in some positive experiences of being together, you've got a powerful, one-two combination. In our experience, if a couple can just get three good days in row—and even better, build on that for ten or twenty—they can usually turn a corner toward a much happier relationship.

EMPATHY

Empathy is the foundation of the experience of "we" rather than just "I" or "you." If you sense that another person really gets how it is for you—or is at least trying to—you'll likely feel less stressed, plus closer and more trusting, and more inclined to be empathic yourself. We are all able to be empathic if we choose; it's an innate human capacity: Even infants are moved by the distress of other babies. Of course, we can have empathy for the good news and happiness of others, though here we will focus on improving empathy for the challenges and stresses of you and your partner, since that often declines after children come along.

Receiving Empathy

Let's start with the understanding you'd like to receive. Other people could give you empathy for both the good and the bad, how life is in general, how it feels to be a mother, and how they affect you. Often, it's the little things that we really want to share: how it felt when your baby—finally!—went to sleep, the humor in a toddler's repeated efforts to hold mashed potatoes in a spoon that's upside down, the frustration of trying to schedule an immediate appointment with the pediatrician for your daughter's umpteenth ear infection. Or it could be something big, like the fact that your own father may need more care, or that you are sick and tired of picking up after everybody else.

Your partner could offer empathy for how you feel worn out, for any health problems you have, for how you might be depleted. You entered a new kind of life when your baby was born and are no longer a free agent, but nested now in a web of connections and obligations that tugs at your every move. You're not saying you want to avoid all that comes with being a mother. But you'd sure like its effects on you to be understood.

You might like empathy for feeling pulled in different directions, such as missing your job while also wanting to stay home, or loving time with your kids while hating housework, or feeling intense compassion for your son in a tantrum combined with an intense desire for him to calm down. You want others to understand that you have ups and downs for reasons, that you're not out of control or weird, that millions of other mothers have similar experiences due to similar causes (see the box).

Research on Mothers

Studies have generally found that:

- Mothers are more emotionally affected by parenthood than fathers.
- Child-rearing and housework are mainly done by mothers, even when both parents work for pay.

- The typical inequities in the total workload make mothers upset, angry, and even depressed.
- A mother often feels pulled in opposing directions by her partner and her children.
- Childcare issues rattle mothers more than fathers, and working mothers experience more stress and overload from juggling both roles than their husbands do. A mother is typically more impacted by her husband's job than he is by hers.
- On average, women experience a sharper drop in marital satisfaction after children than men do. Marital problems wear more on women, who usually place a higher value on relationships and are more economically vulnerable to the impact of divorce.
- A woman is more likely than her partner to be dissatisfied by her marriage, and twice as likely to seek a divorce.

It's in your partner's interest to know how it is for you. It gives him useful information about your inner world, what's really important to you, and the reasons behind your feelings and actions. It's also in his children's interest that he understand you better so you two can work well together, and so his kids can have a mom who feels well nourished in her marriage. He'll be especially able to empathize if you:

- ✦ Talk about your inner world of feelings and longings, not only about the children, events, or your partner.
- ✦ Share your experience in simple, clear terms without justifying or defending it.
- ✦ Speak from your heart.

- Emphasize the softer, deeper, and sometimes "younger" feelings of fear, sadness, hurt, or shame that usually underlie feelings of resentment, disapproval, or anger.
- Speak in the form of *When you do ______, I feel ______*, rather than being accusatory or saying *You* made *me feel ______*.
- Make clear the essence of what you are saying rather than talking around it with euphemisms, hints, word clouds, or detached intellectualizing.

This way of speaking is responsible, open, and dignified. It feels rewarding regardless of your partner's response. Hopefully, he will be understanding, but if he is not, you could directly ask for empathy. It is as legitimate to ask for empathy as it is to ask for help with your child. His empathy is real, even if you have to ask for it. And you can ask him to give you more empathy in general without you having to ask for it!

Of course, he could already be more empathic than you think. As a generalization with exceptions, men tend to view *receiving* empathy as a sign of potential weakness, so they often *give* it indirectly—using action, advice, or joking—as a sign of respect for others . . . such as you. For example, a year into parenthood, Rick was grousing to a friend about his life being turned upside down. Larry had just sent his own son off to college, and he said reassuringly, *Don't worry, it's just a phase. It will be over soon.* Then he smiled and added in his Texas twang, *In about 18 years.* Still, even if his intentions are good, you might like a tone that is more caring and forthcoming, one that envelops you in a warm embrace. You might prefer more words, more details about his understanding of you, more self-disclosure that shows he gets it from the inside out. And whenever you feel his empathy for you, it's good to take a few seconds to let the experience sink in.

Giving Empathy

Now let's take a closer look at giving empathy, because that's something you can each do for your relationship. Also, the more skillful you are at giving empathy, the more you'll know, deep inside, what you can ask for when you'd like your partner to be more empathic with you. In sum, when someone is being empathic, he or she is *paying attention, inquiring,* and *double-checking.*

Paying attention. We can all tell if someone is fully present, rather than thinking about something else, such as their rebuttal. You and your partner can help yourselves be attentive in these ways:

- **Consciously choose to give your attention.** Attention is a gift. See if you can let your partner have your mind, in a sense, for a time. You can take it back whenever you like.
- **Focus on the other person's experience**, the underlying feelings, wants, and thoughts more than the surface details or words.
- **Listen with your body.** Try sensing into your partner's experience from your heart and gut, not just your head.
- **Only listen.** Try not to look for holes in your partner's statements, offer advice, or explain why there's really no reason to get so bothered. The listener's role is simply to understand, without agreeing or disagreeing, approving or disapproving, letting the other person's communications flow without resistance.

Inquiring. Empathy is a process of discovery in which you try to gain an ever-deepening sense of the inner life of another person (for some possible questions, see the box). Through inner reflection and outward inquiry, the empathic partner:

- **Tries to get a sense of the softer feelings**—hurt, fear, sadness, or shame—that lie behind a controlled, tough, or angry facade.
- **Considers the underlying, positive wants** the other person is trying to fulfill—such as desires for closeness, safety, autonomy, or being valued—though perhaps the methods used to achieve these wants are a problem for you.
- **Thinks how the other person's childhood might be a factor today**, and listens for the younger wants and feelings beneath the surface.
- **Imagines the inner being** behind the other's eyes.
- **Listens for the different parts of the other person's experience** so that each can be understood in its own right. For example, if a mother is fuming about her older sister interfering with the 40th wedding anniversary party she is organizing for their parents, one part of her reactions might be feeling overloaded by all the details, another could be resistance to a bossy big sister, and a third part could be a long-standing prickliness about criticism from anybody linked to a childhood with perfectionistic parents. Her partner could try to imagine how each of those parts feels for her, or how they tug at her emotions in different ways.

Empathy Questions

Can you say more about ______________?

What do you mean when you say ______________?

Can you give me an example?

How was it for you that ______________?

How did you feel when they told you about ______________?

Could you say it in a different way so I can understand it?

How irritated were you? (Or worried, hurt, alarmed, sad, etc.)

What was the most upsetting part? (The most annoying? The most worrisome?)

What do you wish would have happened instead?

What do you feel underneath all that?

Did you also feel hurt? (Or embarrassed, ashamed, helpless, etc.)

What does ______________ remind you of?

How does the history of ______________ affect how you feel about ______________?

Deep down, what is really bothering you about ______________?

Double checking. A listener needs to let a speaker know, "Message received." Otherwise, the other person will have to express him- or herself more intensely to get through, or give up and feel unheard. You can show you got the message by saying back, as best you can, both the explicit content and the implicit feelings, wants, and context. If you do this before launching into a reply, your partner is more likely to feel heard even if you have a different point of view.

Empathy for a Father

One of the best ways to encourage your partner to give you empathy is to express it yourself. Here we draw on Rick's experience as a dad and our conversations with fathers to suggest how it may be for him to be a parent; this is a composite, a generalization, of a father that may not fit exactly.

Now I'm a dad. As profoundly as you, he loves the child you are raising together. He has many of the same feelings as you, like happiness when the baby first curls her tiny fingers around one of his own, delight at the first step, and worry over crying that won't stop. And sometimes his sense of things may differ: He might feel less concerned about a knee scraped by a tumble or more embarrassed if your son freezes onstage at the preschool holiday party.

If he spends less time with the children than you, it would be natural for him to be less sure of his skills. Feeling awkward or inept is uncomfortable for many men and makes it hard to ask for help. If you poke fun or criticize him if he does, it gets even harder.

Plunged back into the sights and sounds and smells of childhood, long-forgotten feelings and yearnings from his own early years may be reawakened. That could trouble anyone, but especially a man who is leery of murky or childlike emotions.

Tugged in different directions. He might be showing his love for the children and you in part by stepping up his efforts as a provider. Yet that could draw him into working longer hours when you wish he'd put more energy into your children and home. Unfortunately, his workplace may care little about the needs of his family no matter what the personnel manual says. He could be more engaged in child-rearing and housework than his own father was. Nonetheless, if you are like most mothers, you'd probably like more involvement and help, so he could feel worried and defensive about not coming up to that standard.

The changing, unclear societal expectations about what it is to be a father make it harder to find his footing. There are few cultural models of a man's man who fully shares in parenthood with his wife. Nor is there always respect for the role fathers play in the lives of their children. For example, he has probably had this experience or a similar one: While you're both out in public with your baby, strangers will come up and coo over the baby and you, but mainly ignore him.

Married to a mother. He is probably awed at your ability to make a baby and deeply grateful that you have enabled him to have a child. He probably appreciates the load you've been carrying more than he's been able to say.

He also could be worried by its effects on you, by any fatigue, depression, or other health problems that have developed since you became a mother. He wants you to feel better because he cares about you. But if he offers well-meaning suggestions, such as getting more exercise or using more childcare, you might become irritated, thinking his idea is impractical, wanting empathy rather than problem-solving, or feeling he's trying to get you to give less to your kids. After a few rounds of this, maybe he stops trying.

When it's your turn to offer suggestions, this time about his parenting, he could feel uncomfortable, even annoyed, at being instructed by anyone, especially a woman, especially his wife. As one father told Rick, *Most men wouldn't want their wife to be their boss.* Maybe he's asked you what he could do and been told he should already know. Maybe he's tried to dive in and help and then been told he's doing it wrong. He picks up your underlying attitude about his parenting skills, and the way many mothers talk to each other about their partners is remarkably disdainful. He may experience you squeezing him out of the parent role while complaining that he's not involved enough.

Where did my wife go? He loves his child deeply, and meanwhile, his relationship with you is still a high priority in itself, not merely as a framework for raising children. He (usually) didn't marry a mother and could wonder *Where did my wife go?*

Most of the fathers we've known have felt the loss of attention, affection, and cherishing that have shifted away from them after children come along. While it may be inevitable, it is still a loss. The natural egocentrism of the mommy-baby unit can make a father feel like little more than a means to its ends. One father said: *I go out in the world like a caveman who brings home the meat. I drop it at her feet, she looks up and says thanks, and then goes back to our daughter. It's like I'm not in the room.* Your husband may have had the lurching moment of truth that Rick describes for himself: *One day when Forrest was about a year old, he and Jan were laughing and cuddling on the couch. She smiled at me and I felt her love, but it just landed on me: He was the centerpiece of her life, the sun who lit up her day, not me. I had a jumble of feelings: sadness and loss for myself, bittersweet happiness for Forrest, a sense that this was how it was meant to be, resignation, and acceptance.* If, as Freud thought, there's an Oedipal competition between father and child for the mother, Dad is usually the loser for at least many years. This shift in a mother's caring away from her partner is made painfully concrete by the lack of interest many have in sex (a subject in chapter 8).

Does my partner understand me? A deep question in any important relationship is *Do you really understand me?* And perhaps the deepest question of all is *Do you want to?* Unless each of you can answer yes to both of these questions, they will keep troubling your relationship.

You cannot make your partner understand you, but you can try to understand *him:* That much is in your own power and it increases your chances of receiving understanding in turn. You could ask him about the description of a father just above. Or you could simply observe him for a while without any assumptions, wondering how it feels to be him deep down inside.

With all the caregiving demands in being a mother, you might understandably be feeling some "empathy fatigue." So it may take a conscious decision to bring empathy to your partner. But if you do, there's a good chance that he will notice your interest and appreciate it and be more supportive of you as well. And when you have a better idea of the feelings and wants of each other, you'll be more able to solve problems together.

SPEAKING YOUR MIND

There are surely times to bite your tongue. But holding back your true feelings can lead to a general atmosphere of emotional distance (as well as wear on your health). Family is about closeness if it's about anything. When parents talk to each other mainly from their heads about impersonal matters, that sends a message that it's not desirable or safe to meet in a deeper way. Children notice and become more cautious themselves. You feel stifled, weighted down with what you're holding back. Your partner misses out on important information about how you really think and feel, losing chances to learn and grow. Additionally, you need to be able to openly address any issues in your partner—such as a drinking problem or depression—that affect him, you, or your children.

Again and again, we've seen that the single most beneficial step a couple can take after children is to make deep and open communication a regular and fundamental part of their relationship. By building civility and empathy, you can make it safe enough to be more transparent, vulnerable, and authentic.

In this way of communicating, you are in your experience as you express it. For example, if you were to tell your mate, *I felt disrespected when you criticized me in front of the kids,* you would feel your hurt and anger as you spoke, and he'd hear them in your voice. You would be focused on your own experience and viewpoint, not on getting him to agree or change. You are communicating what you need to say to be true to yourself. There is a lovely sense of freedom and dignity, of being real, of taking care of yourself.

As great as this feels, it's not easy for many of us to speak in this way. For example, you might have grown up hearing instructions such as *If you can't say something nice, don't say anything at all.* As a girl and then a woman and now a mother, you may have thought that your first concern should be the feelings of others, that you shouldn't rock the boat, that you should never get angry or make anyone feel uncomfortable. Simply reflecting about why it might make you nervous to speak your mind fully will help remove any of those soft muzzles over your true voice.

You can also remember the work you've done with your partner to create a safe environment in which you can be vulnerable and real. You can tell yourself that you have a right to your experience and to express it. You do not need to justify your feelings; no one can argue with your description of your own state of mind. Nor do you have to feel that you are stuck with what you say because it's somehow set in stone. In fact, communicating your experience or viewpoint can lead these to flow into becoming something else. And your partner will probably be more open himself if you put your own cards on the table.

POSITIVE SUPPORT

When you and your mate are worn out by raising a family, it's harder to give each other positive energy. But that's when you need acknowledgment and reassurance the most, since researchers have found that receiving emotional support from one's partner is a powerful way to reduce the stress of parenting and increase personal well-being.

Acknowledgment

> *Kind words can be short and easy to speak, but their echoes are truly endless.*
>
> Mother Teresa

After becoming a parent, most people deserve respect, appreciation, and praise more than ever. They're having to learn new things all the time, handle new stresses, and dig deep for love while working day and night. They also need acknowledgment more than ever to compensate for both the Supermom myths that no can live up to and the natural worries about not doing a good enough job in every aspect of life. Unfortunately, people often get fewer positive "social supplies" after they have children. For example, we've seen a mother's partner being too busy to notice, or too worn out or grouchy to say anything, or waiting for a kind word himself.

So it's natural if you'd like to feel more acknowledged by him. One way is to notice his appreciation when it's not stated outright, but sits behind his words or his eyes. Another is to ask for it directly. Some of the most powerful moments in a relationship come when one person is brave enough to ask questions like: *In what ways do you think I am a good mother? A good homemaker? What do you respect about me? What do you see as my strengths? Why do you like me?* You can also ask for more information after he says something, as in: *What did you think was good about the [way I handled that tantrum, thing I said at the teacher's conference, etc.]? Could you be more specific about what you thought I did that worked?*

Yet asking can be hard: Perhaps you were taught to be humble, or you worry that he might laugh or have nothing to say. To overcome these self-doubts, you could remind yourself of all that you do, or consider how it is good for your kids to see him being appreciative. There's a good chance that he'll be large-hearted when you ask him sincerely. If he is not, you will have learned about an issue you need to deal with as a couple. Either way, something good will have happened.

Sometimes we sit down at the banquet table of life, in front of an acknowledgment we have richly earned, and then take only tiny bites, leaving most of it on the plate. Instead, try to treat it as an honest expression of his view of the facts. An acknowledgment is a gift, and it would be rude not to receive it. Even if you think you don't deserve it, he does—and he's probably right.

Turnabout can't hurt either: Giving him acknowledgment both recognizes his efforts and virtues and encourages him to return the favor to you. You could reflect on why you fell in love with him in the first place, on his positive qualities, on the kind soul deep within him, looking out from behind his eyes. When you acknowledge him, you are not ignoring his foibles, but simply recognizing some of the good tiles in the mosaic of the person he is. Unless you have stumbled into a relationship with a really problematic person, the positive tiles greatly outnumber the negative ones. Do your statements about him have roughly the same ratio of positive to negative? You might think back over the last few days: About how many times did you praise or thank him compared to the times you were critical? Besides what you said out loud, how often did you have acknowledging thoughts about him rather than critical ones?

If the balance of your words or thoughts is not consistent with the total mosaic of who your partner is, he could likely feel unseen and misjudged. Meanwhile, this negative tilt could make you feel worse about your relationship than you need to. On the other hand, think of a time when you acknowledged your partner: How did he respond? How did you feel? You might quietly do an experiment for a week of deliberately saying one true thing each day that acknowledges him—and see what happens.

Of course, you are a mosaic yourself, with many more positive characteristics than negative ones. You can certainly ask him to talk about you in a way that is consistent with the total package of who you are, rather than concentrating on the tiles he wishes were different.

Reassurance

If raising a family doesn't make you worry about one thing or another—whether it's a baby who won't stop crying, how to pay the bills, or where a toddler put your car keys—you'd better check your pulse. Strong partners offer reassurance to each other; besides giving it yourself, it is certainly reasonable to ask for it directly, in one or more of these forms:

- *Camaraderie* that you are in this together.
- *Encouragement,* whose root meaning is to give heart. He can remind you of your strengths, of the capabilities you've marshaled before and will call on again. He can look in your eyes and tell you, in his own words, what he knew when you decided to have a child together: *You are a good and strong and capable person, and I believe in you.*
- *Hope* that Mother Nature is on your side, that children eventually learn to sleep through the night, use a toilet on their own, and be nice to each other.
- *Realistic perspectives* about the facts and the risks involved in whatever you are concerned about. He might think that there is less to worry about, or more ways to solve a problem, than you had considered. Of course, this kind of reassurance goes down better *after* he has heard you out, and when it is offered respectfully, without patronizing or dismissing you.

MAKING REPAIRS

Like anything that is precious, fragile, and valuable, a good relationship needs regular maintenance. Within an interaction, couples with a strong relationship make little repairs on the fly, to:

- Clarify intentions
- Correct misunderstandings
- Revise their choice of words
- Drop in grace notes to soothe a ruffled feather

- Lighten the mood by cracking a joke
- Soften a criticism with a self-deprecating admission

And over the long haul, supportive partners act on any sense that there's something festering under the carpet, seeking out and repairing unresolved grievances or misunderstandings.

After years of working with couples, we are convinced that you can almost always find ways to mend what's frayed in any relationship, *if* both partners try hard enough. As we'll see in the next two chapters, there are powerful tools and skills that you can use both as co-parents and as intimate friends, and when you do, these two aspects of your relationship *will* get better.

CHAPTER SEVEN

Partners in Parenthood

If a mother and father do not come together about how to raise their children, there's more stress on the person who handles the bulk of the day-to-day parenting—typically the mother. As well, unresolved disagreements about sharing the load wear most on the person who is doing the majority of the work—again, typically the mother. Besides being personally depleting, these conflicts about raising a family eat away at the bonds that hold a marriage together.* And of course, all this affects children as well.

These can be real problems. Nonetheless, we've seen many people solve them—including in our own relationships—by using the tools in this chapter.

* For simplicity, we'll use "mother," "father," "marriage," and related terms. Still, the material in this chapter could apply to same-gender couples, parents who are divorced, and a parent raising a child with a new partner.

PARENTING FROM THE SAME PAGE

One mother told Rick: *I feel that Angelina, our 4-year-old, should spend only an hour a day on screens. My husband mumbles, "OK, honey," but when I leave the house I come back to see her glued to some screen. I say no sweets, he says just a couple. I say bed by 8, but that means I've got to do it. I read books about parenting that he barely glances at. I'm afraid we are confusing our daughter—plus driving each other crazy!*

It's hard to get on the same page. Parents often have different values or styles in child-rearing. Issues of who gets to be "right" or "in charge" muddy the water. Experts weigh in with conflicting views. Any special concerns about a child—such as health problems or a challenging temperament—strain the parents and their relationship further.

When their parents are working from different "manuals," children get understandably confused. They have to keep switching gears, depending on who they're dealing with. Kids are more likely to play one parent against the other: *But Dad said I could!* And it is disheartening and frustrating if your partner approaches the most important undertaking in your life in a way that to you seems wrongheaded or cavalier.

Minor differences in parenting style are alright. They help children prepare for a variety of teachers, coaches, and (eventually) bosses. Complementary approaches can build on each other, like one parent being more of a tender owie-kisser and the other one an exuberant horseyback-ride-giver, so kids get the best of both worlds. But major differences in parenting values or actions are a problem. To solve it, the first step is to pin down exactly what they are, so we suggest you take a few minutes to reflect on or fill out the questionnaire in the box.

Are We Parenting from the Same Page?

Indicate the degree to which you and your partner agree on the topics below, using this scale:

1 We mainly disagree.
2 We somewhat disagree.
3 We somewhat agree.
4 We mainly agree.

Values: The importance of . . .

________ being sensitive and responsive to your children
________ respecting their wants
________ preventing their discomfort or unhappiness
________ promoting their psychological development
________ accepting and encouraging their self-expression
________ personally interacting with them
________ physical affection toward them
________ their religious upbringing

Actions:

________ Where your children sleep
________ Bedtimes
________ How they are put to bed
________ How you deal with them if they wake up at night
________ How long to breastfeed
________ How many sweets or snacks they are allowed to eat
________ Expectations for their behavior at mealtimes
________ How much screen time they are allowed to have
________ What sorts of TV shows, videos, or movies they see
________ How many toys to buy them
________ Yelling at them when they misbehave
________ Other consequences for misbehavior

________ What to do when a child gets upset

________ How to intervene when siblings quarrel with each other

________ How to intervene when your child quarrels with another child

________ What a parent should do if he or she has made a mistake with a child

Add up your total score. Here is a rough estimate of the degree to which you and your partner parent from the same page (if you skipped some questions, just adjust the ranges below downward):

85–100 Together, you are raising your children in a very consistent way.

70–84 You agree more than you disagree, but there could be some significant differences.

55–69 There are major differences in how you approach child-rearing.

Below 54 Your partner and you are parenting from different books, not just different pages.

Before I got married I had six theories about bringing up children; now I have six children and no theories.

Lord Rochester

Parents often work out their differences informally: Maybe you blurt out something over dinner, there's a testy exchange, one of you makes a point that's too sensible to disagree with, and you come together. But other times, you might benefit from a process that is a little more structured.

Talk About Values

A good place to start is to set aside time to talk about the values that guide your parenting. You can use the questions that follow or come up with your own. This should be an empathic exploration of how each of you feels rather than an attempt to change anyone's mind. Be as supportive as you can and emphasize where you already have common ground. Really try to understand how your partner came to feel the way he does, and you can ask him to do the same for you.

Questions About Parenting Values

Ask your partner these questions and consider them yourself. For example, you could take turns answering one question after another. Feel free to change or eliminate questions as you like. If you are confused by an answer from your partner because it seems different than his actions, you can ask him to clarify, but try to avoid arguing. Take your time; these questions are not always easy to answer, and it could take several conversations to explore them thoroughly.

How you approach being a parent:

What does it mean to you to be a parent?

How has becoming a parent affected you?

If parenthood were a pie divided into four slices—direct child-rearing, housework, coordinating with others (e.g., pediatrician, teacher, relatives, other parents), and providing for the family—how big is each slice for you?

How you want to raise a child:

What do you think are the most important things to give a child the age of our own?

From your own life experiences, what do you feel are important personal characteristics you'd like to see our child develop? What are the top three or four? Is there a number one?

There are three central aspects to parenting: nurturing, encouraging character and achievement, and being an authority figure. Is there one that's most important to you? If a parent can be high, medium, or low on each aspect, how do you think you should be?

What do you wish your mom had done differently? Your dad? How has that affected the kind of parent you want to be?

How did your parents work out their differences in parenting styles? How has that experience affected the ways that you approach working out differences with me?

How does your personality affect your parenting?

Your values in action:

Do any of your values related to raising a family pull in different directions from each other?

How do you feel you have been generally able to act consistently with your values as a parent? How do you feel you have not?

How do you feel you have become more skillful as a parent? How would you like to become more skillful in the future?

Support Each Other

See if you can get agreement on the general goal of supporting each other as parents. For starters, keep each other up to date by sharing information like *I think Charlie's getting a cold* or *Patrice has to bring something to share to kindergarten.* And try to back the authority of the other parent in front of the children whenever possible, handling disagreements behind closed doors with voices that do not fill the home.

Children take their cues for how to treat their parents from seeing how they treat each other, and insulting, hostile, threatening, or raging speech gives children the message that it's alright to speak that way themselves. You both could consider how a child's gender might affect his or her reactions. For example, a boy hearing his father routinely boss his mom around may think that is how men are allowed or even ought to act with women. A girl observing her father act in that way may come to believe that such treatment is normal, and perhaps even unconsciously seek out a man who will treat her similarly when she becomes a woman herself.

You can encourage your children to accept parental authority by going along with it in each other. If Mom calls the family to dinner, Dad should not dawdle. If Dad says it's time to get in the car for a family vacation, that's not the best moment for Mom to make a quick call to a neighbor.

Finally, try not to polarize roles so that one parent is the disciplinarian while the other gets to be more nurturing or playful. This could apply in different ways for each parent. For example, a stay-at-home mom may feel she has to keep redirecting her three-year-old to get through the daily marathon while her partner gets to come home from work with a flashy sprint of high-energy play that kids love. On the other hand, no parent wants to be pegged as the source of big punishments—*Just wait until your father/mother gets home!*—especially if that's a role one of their own parents played. You can talk about this issue and sometimes deliberately shift who does what.

Use a Tie-Breaker

A book, professional, or class is a neutral guide that can break a deadlock between parents. For example, if there's a conflict about how to guide your child's behavior, the two of you could read a credible book on this topic, carve out any parts that either of you does not feel good about, and then use the rest of the book as an agreed-upon "manual" for that aspect of child-rearing. If a big issue comes up—such as you want to try a family bed while he feels the baby should sleep down the hall—the two of you could discuss it with your pediatrician. Many parent resource centers or local therapists offer classes, and taking one together would give you a common experience and an opportunity to hear ideas from other moms and dads.

Informally, you could have another couple over and ask how they handle issues like time-outs or tantrums. This can be reassuring: Behind what appears to be the perfect family is usually a messy reality that may look a lot like your own. Even if you don't get any new techniques, there's the calming sense of perspective that you are grappling with a normal-range problem and that if you hang in there, things will work out like they have for countless other parents. But avoid getting drawn into a fight, whether it's yours—or theirs!

Parenting is still more art than science, but in the last fifty years, much excellent research has established some of the facts of optimal child-rearing; the box summarizes those studies. Disputes can be resolved or at least clarified by finding out what science has discovered about that aspect of raising kids. But keep in mind that many disagreements are fundamentally about values and cannot be resolved by facts alone, that each child is an individual who may differ from the average tendency of the groups that are the basis of most studies, and that any parenting experts who sound completely sure of themselves are probably worth some skepticism.

What Promotes Optimal Child Development

- Good food and health care, a safe environment, and a supportive community
- Many loving and affectionate interactions each day between parent and child
- Sensitive and rapid responsiveness to a child's wants—whether to fulfill them, offer an alternative, or compassionately say no
- A generally positive emotional atmosphere in the home
- Discussion and modeling by parents of character and moral values
- Encouragement to develop age-appropriate skills, including in school
- Clear expectations for developmentally appropriate behavior
- Consistent and appropriate rewards for good behavior and consequences for poor behavior
- No spanking or other corporal punishment
- No harsh, erratic, or abusive parenting practices
- Parents who work together as a strong team

Negotiate Your Differences

Strong couples negotiate all the time, whether it's how to answer a child's fears about sleeping alone in a dark room or what to watch on TV tonight. It doesn't mean you don't love each other if you sometimes find yourselves striking a bargain like shoppers at a flea market. Getting skillful at negotiation can only serve your relationship—plus help you with your child, whether he's two or twenty. These are the six essential steps:

1. Know what you want.
2. Establish a favorable foundation.
3. Communicate clearly.
4. Respect feelings.
5. Work out the details.
6. Make a commitment.

#1 Know what you want. Negotiating is all about wants. To get what you want, you need to know what it is. As we saw in chapter 2, our wants are layered, like a parfait, with less important and fleeting desires on top and vital and enduring ones underneath. The deeper you go, the more you will get to what you *really* want. And the more you and your partner can talk about what you each really want, the more teamwork and friendship you'll have in your relationship.

Therefore, try to probe beneath the surface of your wishes or complaints—such as being peeved that your partner routinely comes home late from work—to find the deeper stakes, which in this case might include wanting to feel that you matter enough to him that he would care about how his lateness affects you, or that you can trust him to keep his agreements. Try to sort the wants from your childhood into a pile that's separate from those that come from a more adult place within your mind. For example, perhaps people kept you frequently waiting as a kid, you hated the boredom and powerlessness of it, and the strong desire to not let that happen again is getting mixed in with your need as a grown woman for him to get home early enough to help you during one of the most stressful times of the day, the mad dash before dinner.

When you acknowledge and accept the child-wants, you'll usually feel a softening inside, and a nurturing kindness toward yourself. You'll also see ways that the situation you faced as a child was different from the one you're in today. That simple understanding has an amazing power to lower the emotional charge on your desire (let's say) for your husband to stop coming home 20 minutes late. When it's time to talk about your wants, it might help to tell him the parts that come from your childhood so he can have a better understanding of what's linked in your mind to seemingly small issues, such as being 20 minutes late. Your openness will probably evoke more compassion and support from him—and if it doesn't, you can ask for it.

Take a close look at any thoughts that argue against your wants, such as *Oh, it's just not practical for him to get home on time every single night.* If the thought has merit, it could lead you to adjust your wishes, like telling your partner that you can live with him coming home late one night in five, or that you just want him to give you a call when he knows he's going to be late. But many thoughts are not good friends to us, as they try to talk us out of wants that are in fact legitimate, reasonable, and positive. Try to challenge those thoughts like this: *Is there really some rule that says I can't ask for that? Would the world come to an end if I got what I wanted? Do other people make the same assumptions when it comes to their own wants?* Another person may not give you what you want, but that does not mean it was bad to want it in the first place, or to express it. For example, as a parent, it is really alright to want the other parent to be more supportive while you are settling a siblings' quarrel. It is OK to want the other parent to use a different tone of voice with your children. It is fine to want the other parent to make some deliberate efforts inside the mind, such as staying mentally and emotionally engaged during a family activity.

#2 Establish a favorable foundation. Try to create a context of mutual rapport, empathy, and good wishes. Choose a good moment and place and be prepared to take the time you need, rather than tossing off comments as you rush on by. Try to frame the issue as a "we" problem rather than an "I" or "you" problem. You are in the same boat together, each affected by the other's actions or suffering. Try to treat each other as respected teammates in a big, challenging, wonderful, and important undertaking.

#3 Communicate clearly. Try to say what you want explicitly and without apology, rather than hinting or saying nothing while hoping the other person will somehow just know. Of course, this can be difficult for several reasons. You may think that what you want should be obvious by now. But it often isn't—especially if your partner is not holding in mind as much information about the kids as you are. It is also common to have had experiences as a child yourself that make it feel scary to really come out with what you want. Using the tools in chapters 2 and 6, try to be aware of those inhibitions. Inside your own mind, challenge the expectations from childhood that are probably not true today, and give yourself encouragement to push forward and let your true voice ring free. (A structured exercise that could support you in expressing your wants is shown in the box.)

Sharing Wants with Your Partner

In this exercise, one partner asks the other one a simple question over and over: *What do you want from me?* Then you switch roles, and the one who was asking the question now starts answering it, over and over. Start by agreeing that you will respect what the other person says and not use it against him or her later. Try to create a context that feels safe.

As a questioner, all you need to do is ask the question genuinely and listen empathically to the answer. Do not comment or criticize, although you can ask your partner to clarify something you don't understand. After he has answered, say *I got it* or something similar, and ask the question again.

As a speaker, look inside each time you hear the question and see what else you want from your partner. It is fine to express wishes that seem whimsical, silly, embarrassing, or taboo; you are only sharing your experience in the moment, not committing to a position. You are trying to open the whole bag onto the table, including wants that are general *(that you act more loving)* and specific *(that you put the cap on the toothpaste).* It is alright to express wants that come from the younger parts of yourself, including those that are more about your own parents than your partner. Try to push through any holding back and say what you really long for, whatever it is.

Set aside half an hour or more to do this exercise. Try to get through at least a dozen rounds of questions per person. If you each can, let yourselves go into a deep place of honesty and intimacy with each other. Afterward, talk about the exercise, but do not argue about it.

If you'd like, alter the form slightly by having the questioner respond to each answer by saying either *Yes, I can do that* or *Let's talk more about it.* You can also use this format with related questions, such as: *What would you like for our family? What do you need from me to trust me? What are you afraid of? What is bothering you? How could I be a better partner?*

Once you start talking, try to explain your point of view in terms that will make sense to the other person, given *their* values and concerns. Avoid distractions such as other issues or arguing about what happened in the past. Anticipate objections and doubts. You can make it easier to try the approach you're suggesting by framing it as an experiment, putting a time limit on how long you'll give it a go, and perhaps linking it to certain conditions: *Could we just try for a week insisting that Serena eat some vegetables before dessert and see what happens, and if she goes on a hunger strike, we can do something else?*

It's especially useful to translate general wants into concrete specifics, using examples of how things will be if you get what you want. This brings issues down out of the clouds of abstractions like "spoiling children" to solid ground where you can actually *do* something. It lets your partner know exactly what you'd like him to do, and it enables you to know if it gets done. For example, instead of saying *You're too permissive,* try *I think you let the kids have too many sweets. I'm willing for the kids to have dessert at dinner but not a candy bar in the afternoon, too. OK?* Overall, focus on positive behaviors by saying what you want more of rather than less.

Of course, it's also alright to be clear about where you are unclear: *I think we ought to try a new babysitter but I'm not 100 percent convinced—what do you think?* Or *I feel like we need to push harder on toilet training, but I'm not sure how to do it; do you have any ideas?*

To be sure, you need to find out what he wants, so you have to ask or give him the space to say it. If it is not obvious, try to get at the wish or complaint embedded in his communication. Don't shy away from differences. Sometimes a couple will avoid conflicts by ignoring their issues, but the result is a tepid, distant relationship that is just not anchored in truth. The issues will come boiling out one day, anyway, or some passing gust of wind—an unexpected pregnancy, a layoff at work—could blow the relationship away like a tumbleweed with no roots. Ask questions even if you fear the answers: *What is really bothering you? What's the most important part of this to you? What would make things better? What would it look like if you got what you want?* It is OK to discover that your partner wants something from you that you do not want to give; it is really alright if he does not love every single thing about you or approve of everything you do; you cannot please him—or any person—all of the time.

Finally, prevent miscommunications before they happen by double-checking. You could ask what he thinks you want. Or you could tell him what you think he wants. These simple steps are amazingly effective in creating a solid foundation of mutual understanding.

#4 Respect feelings. Communicating wants often brings up feelings, some of which can go all the way back to our childhood. If these are not acknowledged, they will clamor more loudly, like a child raising her voice to be heard. If you are nervous or irritated underneath, try to say so, because your partner is probably sensing your disquiet and may react to it instead of the topic you want to focus on. For example: *I'm a little nervous about bringing this up, but I don't think our childcare is working out.* Or: *I'm getting frustrated that Evelyn is still crying most times you wash her hair.* Explain why your wants are important to you and how they are linked to your values, and try to find out the same about him. If emotions are clouding your discussion, you may need to shift gears to talking about your feelings for a while, and then get back to negotiating practical arrangements.

#5 Work out the details. Adopt a mindset in which you are moving toward positive solutions instead of wrangling about negative problems. Consider, at least to yourself, any payoff you might be receiving from the current situation—such as getting to feel morally superior or like a virtuous victim—and next consider the costs of that, and then decide what you really want. Study the times when all goes well as a model of what you each can do to make things work. You and your partner could ask yourselves, *What would it be like to no longer have this problem?*

Push to narrow your differences: *It's not that I'm a control freak or you're a hippie, it's that I think Latrell is old enough to put away his clothes and you don't.* Or even closer together: *Can't we just insist that he put his coat on the hook when he gets home instead of dropping it on the floor?* Since people in conflict usually overestimate their differences, chances are that you're closer together than you think. It's a lot easier to bridge a smaller gap.

Sometimes in the throes of a negotiation (or argument), you start to realize that you might be able to live with some difference in parenting style. It's often worth asking yourself questions such as these: *Is it that big a deal? Is it really harming my kids? Is it worth straining my marriage or stressing myself out?* Seemingly opposing practices might in fact be complementary, such as how being highly nurturing to a child promotes independence, rather than dependence, by giving her the sense of a safe base from which she can explore. Maybe it's alright for one parent to put a higher priority on something than the other parent does—like being more zealous about good manners at the table—as long as you don't undermine each other: *It's OK that I don't care about this as much as you do, but I won't get in your way, and I'll support you when I can.* Different approaches can often coexist; it's not the end of the world if the kids know that one parent is a softer touch for a cookie or an extra bedtime story.

Another way to live with differences in parenting is to agree that each partner has veto power if he or she feels strongly about an issue, such as risks to a child's safety. Of course, no one should abuse the veto, and you can take back that power if it gets out of hand.

If important conflicts remain, be willing to make a deal. Consider offering a compromise, or budging on one of your priorities if he gives in on one of his. For example, you could agree for your values to rule in one area while his prevail in another: *I'll loosen up about what the kids wear if you promise to be stricter about bedtimes.* Or find out what parts of an overall task that he might prefer, and see if it works for you to do the other parts.

Try to anticipate potential problems and then pre-solve them. It's not pessimistic to think about what might go wrong; it's reasonable and responsible. By planning together, you and your partner can create a sense of shared confidence in handling whatever comes up.

Last, you can ask yourself: *What could I do that would make it more likely that he will give me what I'm asking for? And what could he do that would help me give him more of what he is asking for?*

#6 Make a commitment. When there is a clear understanding of what you and your partner are going to do, check your gut feeling. Do you and he really think this is going to happen? Or are you kidding yourselves? If your plan feels solid, treat it as a personal commitment and ask him to do the same. You are each giving your word, and that is not a thing to be taken lightly. Then acknowledge the process you have gone through. It's not easy to work out issues in parenting, yet you've each stuck with it.

Finally, try to avoid snatching defeat from the jaws of victory. You may have seen some of the ways this can happen, such as not noticing it when your partner has come over to your side, continuing to hammer your point after they have agreed with you, remaining irritated that you had to talk about it in the first place, or shifting with hardly a breath to another issue.

Talk About Misunderstandings or Broken Agreements

Fulfilling commitments is the basis of trust in any relationship. Nonetheless, no person manages to keep every agreement every single time. Maintaining trust requires communicating when an agreement is broken. If you did not do what you said you would do, try to bring up the matter yourself. Say if this was a onetime event that does not reflect your true intentions. Or explain that you think the plan is unworkable and should be revised.

If it is your partner who departs from the plan, talk about it openly, since silence on your part can be taken as tacit approval. Plus, you need to know what is going on. Perhaps there was ambiguity in the original arrangement, or maybe you misunderstood something and he actually did what he agreed to. Or it could in fact have been a broken agreement. If so, perhaps it was just a temporary lapse and he's back on track. But you may discover that you need to do some more negotiating.

Even though they can be uncomfortable to discuss, if you do not talk about misunderstandings and broken agreements, they will happen again. In particular, if your partner is often flaky or unreliable, if he does not seem willing to make the most fundamental commitment of all—*I agree to keep my agreements*—you've *got* to talk about it. You are entitled to bring a moral seriousness to the discussion, to confront broken agreements for what they are: breaches of trust that erode the foundation of any important relationship. If he says something like *You can't pin me down so much; things change,* a possible reply could be *If you had a colleague at work who said one thing but did another as often as you do at home, how would you feel and what would you do? You would probably feel let down and frustrated, and you would tell the person that there needed to be changes in the way he/she was acting. It's the same here.*

If talking together doesn't work, consider involving a professional such as a therapist or clergy member. Besides letting your partner know you're serious, the thought of airing dirty laundry in front of another person could be enough to prompt a change in behavior. More than once, Rick has made a first appointment with a mother for couples counseling only to receive a second call a few days later canceling the session because *When I told him I'd made the appointment, he finally realized I was really serious, and that's led to some good conversations and changes.* Whatever works!

SHARING THE LOAD

The amount of mental and physical work required to raise a family is staggering, whether it's painting your baby's bedroom or—18 years later—helping her pack for college. Without supportive communities, the work of raising children mainly lands on the two parents alone, pushing them into Condition Yellow even when they have a strong partnership. If either does less than his or her share, the other one is shoved toward Condition Red: more to do, less time to sleep or eat, more dismay and resentment and anger. Compounding things, the parent who is dropping one end of the log may have the audacity to wonder, "Why don't we ever talk/go to the movies/make love anymore?"

Many couples share equally the work of making a family, handling Condition Yellow with tenacity, skill, and grace. But that's the exception, and the rule tilts mainly against women:

- **Tasks:** On average, a mother is working one way or another many hours more each week than the father of her children, whether or not she is drawing a paycheck. An extra hour in the morning, an hour at night, a few hours on each weekend day . . . it adds up pretty fast. Even when a mother makes as much money as or more than her husband, typically she still does more housework and childcare.
- **Emotion work:** This part of making a family may not look like much on the outside, but it is often the most draining. It includes settling squabbles between siblings, worrying about a fever that won't break, or comforting a child who's being picked on at school. Women do most of the emotion work

in families, much as they do in relationships in general. For instance, when both parents are in the room, it is the mother who is most likely to be emotionally available to their child, rather than being engaged with other things such as going over the bills, reading emails, or watching TV.

- **Stresses:** Since tending to young children is more stressful than most jobs, if Mom stays home while Dad goes off to work, her day is usually more stressful than his. When both parents are home, even if each of them spends about the same amount of time doing tasks, the mother typically does the high-stress ones while the father does more peaceful projects he can schedule at will and carry to completion. And when there is nothing left for her to do, a mother often feels stressfully vigilant and on call at a moment's notice, while her partner is more likely to do his tasks and then relax.
- **Responsibilities:** Children live in your heart and weigh on your mind. The consequences of your decisions can be monumental: literally, the health and welfare of an innocent child. For all the advances in the workplace for women over the past fifty years, little has changed at the "Board of Directors" level in most families: It is still usually Mom, not Dad, who does most of the planning, worrying, and problem-solving about the children. It's lonely at the top of the typical family.

> *If evolution works, how come mothers have only two hands?*
>
> Ed Dussault

These inequities impact the children: Studies have shown that fathers who are less involved tend to have kids who are less responsible, less able to solve problems, and less confident, and have lower self-esteem. Inequities also eat away at a marriage, reducing the satisfaction of each spouse. And they deplete a mother, increasing her stress, giving her less time to recharge her batteries, and lowering her mood. As one mother told Jan: *I did all the planning and organizing for Oliver's birthday, thinking that his father would help out during the party itself. But no, he stood around the whole time talking with his buddies while I raced around doing everything, except for when he cut the cake and then looked at me like he deserved some kind of reward! I want someone who doesn't need me to raise my voice to get some help, who takes initiative with the kids and the house, whose mind is not elsewhere all the time. Somebody who does things because he* wants *to do his share, not just to get me off his back. I need to really feel like I have another half.*

And lapses in sharing the load aren't good for a father, either. Avoiding the nitty-gritty tasks of tending to young children—such as changing diapers—can make a father feel less connected, competent, or satisfied with parenthood. Picking and choosing his part of the total load puts him half-in with his family but also half-out, like the man who stood on a dock considering whether to get on a boat. He decided to put one foot on it as a test. At first, everything went fine. But the boat began to move slowly away—one foot, two, three, four—and his legs started to hurt. He thought to himself, "If it feels this bad to put just one foot on that boat, two would be awful," and he jumped back onto the dock. But when a father strides onto that boat as a cocaptain, and he weathers some storms and learns to steer it well, his experience of family life is deeply fulfilling.

It is fine to do different things, such as Mom puts in a load of laundry while Dad gives their kids a bath. But significant unfairness poisons the well of a family. The *why* of sharing the load fairly is clear. The real question is *how*—and here are some suggestions for common situations in which the father could share more of the load.

Clear Facts

The place to begin is to establish what the facts are. Many fathers believe they are doing more than they actually are. For example, even in dual-earner couples, many fathers feel they're doing their fair share of child-rearing, yet in surveys, mothers consistently report carrying more of the load.

Therefore, if there is any question about what is actually happening, we suggest that each of you (or you alone, if necessary) track, for at least a few days and ideally for a week, who does what and for how much time. Each day, just jot down how you spent your time. One way to do this easily is on daily copies of a simple form you can create in which the rows are 15-minute intervals and the columns are different kinds of activities such as interacting with a child or doing housework (or both at the same time!); you can create the form by hand or make a spreadsheet or use a time-tracker app. Additionally, you could each make note of the stresses you experienced that day as well as the sense of responsibility you felt for planning, worrying, and problem-solving.

Alternatively, each of you could simply list what you did with the kids or household that day. If even that would be overwhelming—since the typical mom does several hundred such tasks daily—make a list for an hour or for a specific part of the day such as the morning or evening.

At night, compare notes, and see if you can agree on the basic facts of that day without nitpicking whether something took 5 minutes or 10. At the end of the period, try to agree on what the facts are, plus or minus 10 percent. If you can't, consider involving a third party such as a therapist.

If your partner suddenly becomes an angel once the spotlight is on, you could comment on that. You could also suggest continuing to track time for a few more weeks, which would have one of three outcomes, all of which are good: (1) You might discover that you've had a better partner than you thought, (2) his true colors would be revealed over time if he could not sustain the miraculous transformation, or (3) what started as an exercise in looking good could become a habit.

But in the usual case, people remain more or less true to form, and the results on paper are eye-opening. Rick once worked with a couple in which the mom felt overworked, but the dad thought she was exaggerating because she was mad he was putting so much time into his hobby of music. They tracked their time for a week and saw in black and white that he averaged one hour of sleep and two hours of personal time more than she did each day—which added up to 21 hours a week and over a thousand hours a year of more sleep and personal time for him than her. He couldn't ignore that difference or justify it, so he started spending more time with their child.

Clear Principles

Even with clear facts, parents can disagree about what they *mean*. Cultural factors influence our expectations about the proper sharing of roles after children arrive. In some regions of the country, or within certain groups, it is common to find support for a view of family life in which the woman does most of the childcare and housework, and she may defer to her husband in other matters as well.

Psychological factors also determine how we share the load. A father's active involvement with childcare depends in part on his enjoyment of parenting, his beliefs about the importance of fathers to children, and his feeling that masculine men can be skillful with little kids. The amounts and kinds of housework he does are shaped by his ideas about the fundamental equality of the sexes. You can influence him as well, through your expectations and willingness to assert yourself. But speaking your mind can be hard if you:

- Believe in traditional gender roles
- Think that making money counts for more than childcare or housework, or feel one-down in the relationship because he makes more money than you
- Fear he might leave you or take his anger out on the children
- Feel guilty about pursuing your own career and try to compensate by going overboard on childcare and housework
- Are embarrassed about asking for help, perhaps thinking it makes you look needy, or that you should be able to handle everything on your own
- Think he'll do it all wrong, or feel territorial about your role

Biology plays a part as well. Men vary in their innate interest in child-rearing, much like women do, but to a greater degree. For some perspective, consider that males do next to nothing for their young in 95 percent of the mammal species, including the primates that are our close relatives. "Mating effort"—sowing seeds far and wide—is in most species a more effective reproductive strategy for males than "parental investment," the strategy usually used by females for passing on their genes.

Our species seems to have evolved a mixed strategy in which both inclinations—mating effort and parental investment—interact with each other, and the relative weight of each varies from man to man. We make these points about biology not to let fathers off the hook, but to highlight the poignant reality that is the backdrop of many domestic disputes. That way, you can take your partner's natural inclinations less personally—wherever they are in the range of men—and have compassion and respect for the ways he's trying to work with them. The balance of power in a father between mating effort and parental investment is greatly affected by social and psychological factors. He can help himself by spending time with other dads who are deeply involved with their children, participating in groups or activities that support engaged fatherhood, or reflecting on his ethical duty to his children and their mother. He could apply the same ideals of learning and competence that he lives by at work to his parenting. He might reflect on his relationship with his own father, both what he gained from his dad and how he might like to parent in some different ways, perhaps using the exercise in the box.

A Man's Reflections on His Own Father

In addition to thinking about the following questions, you might like to discuss them with your wife. You could also write your answers as a letter to your father that you will probably never send.

When you were a boy, what was your father's role in the family?

How was your father there for you? How was he not?

Did he spend so much time at work that you felt his job was more important to him than you?

How might he have affected how your mother acted toward you or your brothers or sisters? Did he help her be a good mother? Or did he make her job harder?

What are the ways that you are glad that you are acting like him? Are there any ways you are acting like him that you wish you were not?

What are the ways that you are glad you are not *acting like him? Are there any ways you are not acting like him that you wish you were?*

How do you think your own children will think about you when they are reflecting on their dad like you are today?

You can encourage a father's involvement by helping him see what a difference he makes to his children. You can point out models of masculine-and-competent fathers—including him! Or do little things to help parenting be enjoyable for him, like having him come see your son with his hair shampooed up like a rooster's comb.

In the end, no matter what the cultural, psychological, or biological forces may be in our lives, we still have to make choices based on principle. You have the right to make a case for certain values, to say what you think your children need, and to name what you feel is fair or unfair. Here are examples of principled responses to various objections we've heard fathers make to carrying more of the total load; please adapt them to your own needs and voice:

- *"I'm not as good at it as you are. Plus the kids go to you anyway."*—Like anything, you just need to practice a little. The kids will get used to you doing certain things, and I'll direct them to you more. Plus you could initiate and not wait for the kids to come to me. Additionally, even if I'm the one who always washes Angel's hair, you could still step in more by reading to Michael or cleaning up after dinner.
- *"You always interfere, and I've quit trying."* I don't *always* interfere, but I do sometimes. I'm trying to help, anyway, not interfere, but I can understand that you feel crowded, so I'll promise to back off.
- *"You just want someone to do things for you."* Nope, I want you to do things *with* me. It's not just about getting stuff done. When you do your part, it makes me feel connected to you, like I'm not alone and we're in this together. I made a baby *with* you and I would love for us to share that experience in a happy way together.

- *"I do more than my dad did."* That's great, and I appreciate it. But there is still more to do if we're going to be fair about it.
- *"My job is so stressful that I need to rest at home."* Remember how you nearly fainted with relief when I finally got home after you were alone with the kids that one time for a few hours? Now imagine doing that for many hours instead of a few, and for a thousand days instead of one. If we're talking about getting a break based on the stress level of our typical day, in fairness I deserve rest at least as much as you.
- *"Making a living counts for more than raising children."* I believe that it's the other way around. Child-rearing counts for more since it so directly impacts our precious children. And it's usually harder, day after day. I am not setting child-rearing above making a living. But it is at least equal.
- *"I make all the money, so you should handle the housework and kids."* I *do* handle the housework and kids while you are making money. I'm talking about what you do when you're not commuting or at work. You wanted children and now we've got them. You can see that it's best for them when we are both involved in the morning, at night, and over the weekend. It is not fair for me to keep on going while you watch TV or go out with your friends. How would you feel about someone at work who did that sort of thing while you kept getting things done? Wouldn't you want them to do their share?
- *"I make more money than you."* I appreciate all the money you bring into our family. But that does not change what is good for our children and our relationship when we are both at home in the mornings, evenings, and weekends. (And follow with the points just above.) Additionally, you have the time to make that money because of the work I do at home.

- *"It's because you've got a job that the kids need so much and there's so much housework."* That's hitting below the belt. If I didn't work, our kids would still need you to do your share in the mornings, evenings, and weekends. We need my salary, and even if we didn't, I have as much right to work as you do. Besides, we could just as well turn the point against you: The kids wouldn't need so much if you, their father, stayed home. In fairness, the hard choices between career and time with children should fall just as much on a father as a mother. We both work, we both need to parent, and we both need to do housework.
- *"That's women's work."* There is no law that says so. You did dishes before you met me, and it wasn't women's work then. You don't take it easy out of high moral principle while I wash clothes or give the kids a bath, but simply because that's your personal preference. You're just as capable as I am of putting a child to sleep or feeding a toddler.
- *"Quit telling me what to do."* I don't *want* to tell you what to do. Usually I try not to. And if I ever do, it's because you won't make a reasonable agreement with me about who does what—or you make one but don't stick with it. I'm the messenger of what our kids or home needs, so please don't be angry at me for just bringing that message. If you stepped in to do what needed doing in the first place, I wouldn't have to bring a message at all. Besides, why is it fair for you to tell me what to do about the car/computer/mutual fund/whatever but I can't tell you anything about what to put in a lunch box?
- *"Get off my back, or else."* I'd be glad to talk about this when you're calmer. But I'm going to ask: What's the "or else"? Are you really going to walk out on your kids because I'm tired

of picking up your socks off the floor? Because I'd appreciate it if you'd get home sooner? Your kids need you to be more involved, I need it, and our marriage does, too.

Clear Agreements

Once you come together on basic principles, agreements about actions are more straightforward, especially when you use the negotiation skills we've previously covered. Here are some practical solutions that have helped many families, including those in which the parents are already sharing the load fairly and the remaining need is just how to work together even better.

Apply organizational principles. A family is an organization, and many of the same approaches used in other organizations will work in your home as well. First, you could create a base schedule that guides your week, knowing that you can change it as needed. In it, build in breaks that are fair for each of you. One dad said to Rick: *My wife gets Wednesday night "off" while I take care of the kids. I'll get up early on Saturday morning and go for a hike with a buddy, getting back by noon or so. I think about that hike all week, like she thinks about what she'll do Wednesday night. It's a lifesaver.*

But be sure to take your break when it comes! Many mothers feel like they have to overcome an invisible gravitational field to lift out of their orbit around their children. Remember that you deserve and need this time to yourself, and that your children will benefit from a reinvigorated mother when you get back. You might also arrange to take some of your time off *with* your kids as long as your husband assumes the major responsibility for caring for them. For example, when their kids were young, Rick's idea of a dream vacation was a rock-climbing trip that wasn't possible with their children, while Jan's was a week in the sun somewhere with their children nearby while Rick watched them.

Second, we suggest you distinguish between *responsibility*, which you both share for the family's overall well-being, and individual *accountability* for specific tasks. Then create a basic understanding of what you are each accountable for: Who does what when? You could write it down, and if you have to, post it. Just walk through your day mentally and think about what would help things go well. Could you get the kids dressed while he showers, and then he feeds them while you shower? Would he rather clean up after dinner or put them to bed? Should you pick up takeout on Tuesday night? The details are usually not that hard; much of it is just being good roommates.

Coordinate with each other. Check in before making plans. Rick and Jan got their first big lesson in this just a few months after their first child was born, and Jan describes what happened: *Our good friend Bob was coming to visit, and Rick told me that they were going sailing Saturday. I was dead tired already and asked in disbelief, "You're going to leave me home alone for a day with a baby while you play around?" Rick was startled. In the past, he'd go off with a friend while I did something else with my own friends, and it was no big deal. But now what he did really affected the baby and me, and he had to take* us *into account. He took a long, slow breath and it was like a light bulb went on for him. Then he said, "You're right. Now I need to* ask*."*

Keep things in perspective. It's the overall performance that matters. Nobody's perfect, and overreacting to small lapses can undermine a general spirit of cooperation. Let people do housework their own way; unless dishes are getting broken each night, don't hassle each other about how to load the dishwasher. As a general rule, let the person who is doing the task be in charge of how it gets done.

You can be flexible and creative for the greater good. If he suggests paper plates for most weeknights, maybe that's not so crazy. Perhaps you both can live with a semi-messy kitchen until Saturday morning, when you spend an hour together cleaning it up, drinking some coffee, and talking.

Children are passionately unpredictable in their nature, so it's a good idea to cut each other some slack if some plans go awry. For example, a mother told this story: *We were going somewhere, and I was getting Marion ready while Frank was on the phone. He came in and snapped at me because we were running late. He hates that, and he is Mr. Punctuality at work. But a child doesn't always follow a schedule. He should know that, because if he's the one trying to get her to cooperate, we never leave on time!* Or perhaps step in and help out instead of judging the other parent's performance.

It's alright for you to take the lead sometimes. Unless the mother and father truly share all aspects of parenting equally, more often than not it is the mother who is more actively engaged with the children. Consequently, her partner could be entering a flow of activities that she's been managing, and he is just being a good team player when he asks her, the quarterback, what the play is. In the moment, you can say what you'd like him to do. Later on, if you like, you could talk together about similar situations in the future and figure out what he could do in them without you having to say anything.

Look for ways to support his relationship with the children. If he is hanging back, you could invite him to share in the fun moments, not just the chores. He could think about the interests he'd like to share with his kids, like a love of the outdoors, or the values he wants to help them develop. For instance, reading certain stories to them would be a way to talk about similar experiences he has had or what he thinks is really important in life.

He might say that he'll get more involved when the kids are older and it feels more "natural." This may well be true, and meanwhile he could do more housework while you do more tending to the baby. On the other hand, your child's life is still going on, and he may need to get comfortable with changing diapers ahead of schedule. If so, practice is key, often accomplished by leaving him with the baby for a while and letting him figure things out. You could have another couple over for dinner in which the dad is good with little kids so your mate can see another man act in that way. There is no good reason why someone who can do whatever he does at work all day can't skillfully and lovingly manage a young child.

You may also have to deal with any tendency in your partner to pull back from the kids because he's upset with you. Men are more likely than women to let their relationship with their children be affected by their feelings about their spouse. Doing the right thing by his kids is ultimately up to him, but you can help in several ways. Tell him how much the kids need him no matter what he thinks right now about you. Without walking on eggshells, you could choose to let go of little things to keep the peace. And if you need to, you could play hardball, asking questions like *Do you think a man should walk away from a responsibility just because it's hard or he feels ticked off at a coworker? When our kids are older, what will* they *wish you had done?*

Work out housework issues. One mother said, *He comes home from work and expects the house to look immaculate. I just don't care as much as he does, and even if I did, I would have to follow behind the kids every minute.* On the other hand, a father commented, *She thinks it's her house, that she has some kind of God-given wisdom about it because she's a woman. She freaks out if the dishes are not immediately done after dinner. She literally cannot sit still at the table and relax and talk if there's a dirty glass in the sink.* A few suggestions: Agree to lower your standards while kids are little. Try to keep one room as an orderly sanctuary. In age-appropriate ways, call on your kids to pick up after themselves.

Tackle high-stress situations together. For instance, analyze the morning madness. It all starts the night before, so perhaps he could promise to quit extending your daughter's bedtime with extra stories even though she loves them. Later that night, you could lay out her clothes while he sets up for breakfast. Maybe wake up 15 minutes earlier to have a moment for yourself and a chance to get ready for the day. He could get your child into the car while you finish dressing. And off you all go.

In particular, pay special attention to working well together on any issues with your child, such as a challenging temperament. Try to talk about the different meanings that the situation may have for each of you. For instance, the parent who is more directly involved with child-rearing—typically the mother—might feel that a child's issues are somehow her fault. Together, you could read a book about child development and the particular issue. Try to make a clear plan together that will effectively address your child's needs; if you can't do this on your own, you could get a consultant or tie-breaker.

Balance the total stress load more or less evenly. Try to take into account the nature of each parent's job, the age and temperament of the children, and any other circumstances that pile on stress. Notice if one parent lets the other one handle the stressful jobs, or if one parent automatically jumps in first. For example, does Parent A walk through the door and immediately dive in to settling a squabble or doing a load of laundry while Parent B goes off to change clothes or look through the mail? Maybe Parent A could relax a bit first while Parent B takes more initiative with the kids and the housework.

If he slides into fun jobs with the kids like reading stories while you fold laundry or figure out the checkbook, that could be a break for you from mommy-mode, but it could also mean that you're getting stuck with more than your share of the housework, which might feel boring, unpleasant, and even depressing. To deal with this, try divvying up household tasks, including paperwork, coordinating with others (such as planning a birthday party), maintenance (Who stays home to wait for the plumber?), and yardwork. You could make a list of the major tasks in one column. Then add two other columns, one for each of you, and mark who gets which job. Factor in that some jobs take longer or are worse than others (toilets . . .), consider alternating jobs (if it's an odd day, he does the dishes), and create something that's reasonably fair. If there's an impasse, you can flip a coin. Worst case, you could go on strike and not do a particular job until there's some resolution. This would mean letting go of any compulsion you feel about it, while remembering that he may not feel compelled, and that household tasks are not life-and-death matters.

Address the impact of work on your family. It's very challenging if you both work full-time and get home around 6:00 or later to a mad flurry of activities ending in a collapse in bed. (Unfortunately and unfairly, the effects of the two-career family are commonly framed to blame women when, in principle, a man could as readily scale back his career.) Or one parent might work part-time or not at all while the other one puts in 60 or 70 hours each week, including commuting, business travel, and doing texts and emails from home. When children are young, it's more often the father with the big time-consuming job. That could be one way he fulfills his sense of responsibility to you and the children, but some men use their work to hide from their family. Even with the best of motives, his big job is like an elephant in the living room, limiting the space that's left for everyone else. In that situation, children can grow up with a subtle sense of fatherlessness. Meanwhile, the dad misses out on a special time that will never be repeated, trading it for career moves that often could be postponed a few years. The mom becomes a de facto single parent. And it is hard to work around the elephant to maintain a deeply intimate marriage.

Sometimes absolutely nothing can be done about the jobs you each have. The best you can do then is to try to reduce your other stresses (e.g., lower your standards for housework, don't take on another puppy), increase your resources (such as hiring a neighborhood kid to do some yardwork), and improve your psychological coping (see the tools discussed in chapters 2 and 3).

Usually, though, you *can* do something about your circumstances, especially if you persist. Let's use the example of him working long hours while you stay home with a young child. The first step is to create a positive atmosphere for tackling the issue, approaching it as a "we problem" with no bad guy. For instance, you could express your respect for how hard he works to provide for his family and your understanding that his career is very important to him. Second, challenge the assumptions that box you in. For example, you might consider going back to (perhaps part-time) work ahead of schedule so there is less financial demand for his source of income and therefore more potential options regarding it. For his part, he could do some soul-searching about:

- How this time with children is fleeting and unique, and worth making a special effort to spend with them
- How his children, wife, or marriage would benefit if he were home more; how he would benefit himself
- The beliefs that make him feel embarrassed about saying he needs to leave work at a certain time to get home for his family, or the ways he may be getting caught up in a workplace culture that prides itself on extreme hours
- The extra time he might be spending for work that's about personal rewards distinct from the financial needs of family; personal fulfillment is a valid aim, but it's not selfless sacrifice
- How a small reduction in his time at work—say 10 percent—could have little effect on his career while potentially doubling or tripling his time with his kids—the epitome of a highly leveraged investment!

A rich child often sits in a poor mother's lap.

Danish proverb

Third, you can make a long-term plan that is consistent with your values and is financially realistic. If your circumstances allow this option, your overall quality of life might improve if you spent less money in some ways so you could spend more *time* with each other. The questions in the box can help clarify the values that shape these choices.

Your Values for Life and Money

Please consider these questions:

- *Imagine looking back on your life at age 80 or so: What will you be most glad about, and what will not have mattered much? From that perspective, how will you wish that you had approached money and career?*
- *Imagine that you have one year to live: What would your priorities be? Are there ways to be truer to these priorities if you were to live for 50 more years?*
- *What's your preferred pace of living? How important to you are relaxation and leisure compared to accomplishment, status, and possessions?*
- *How much do you value time with your children, especially while they are young, compared to furthering your career or making money? Given that value, how would you feel about reducing your rate of saving for retirement during the next few years while your children are little?*

- *What's your bottom-line limit on the number of hours each week you want your spouse or yourself to give to work (including commuting and business travel)?*
- *At this time, what standard of living are you determined to have, from weekly spending on lunches out to big-ticket items like major vacations or remodeling your home? What standard of living do you want to have in a few years?*

Unnecessary fears drive many financial decisions, and the antidote is clarity about money and the specific facts of your current expenses and future needs. It's not that hard to create a realistic long-term financial plan that will help you with understanding and prioritizing. Books and websites can guide you through the details. On your own in an hour or less, you could probably come up with a family budget that is accurate within 10 percent. Estimating your needs down the road is more complicated, so it's wise to use a good book or a financial planner, especially if you and your partner disagree about priorities or methods. But with less effort than it took to equip your baby's bedroom, you can likely come up with a realistic plan that makes your jobs serve you and your family, rather than the other way around.

CHAPTER EIGHT

Staying Intimate Friends After Children

Raising children together can nurture a relationship in many ways. Doing things as a family—playing a game, going to the park, making popcorn—creates a circle of love that includes your mate as well as your children. When things get hard, as they do for every couple, having children can motivate partners to dig down and do the work necessary to maintain a strong relationship. Nonetheless, children innocently yet inevitably bring consequences that tend to nudge their mom and dad apart, such as fatigue and depletion, conflicts over child-rearing and sharing the load, and less time to be together as mates. It's so easy for a little more distance to come between you each day, a little more irritation or disdain.

> *We're too busy being parents to be friends.*
>
> A mother

That's why appreciating, protecting, and nurturing your relationship is so important after kids come along. Staying intimate friends helps you feel cherished and secure. It lifts your mood; brings you companionship, affection, and romance; and even bolsters your resistance to illness. And it naturally evokes more consideration, compassion, and help from your partner, and makes it easier to stay out of nasty quarrels.

A strong and enduring love between parents casts a light and a warmth that envelops their children as well. Even when very young, children can sense the quality of feeling between their mother and father. Visible friendship, love, and passion between parents makes children feel secure. And it gives them hope, when they're older, for their own dreams of lasting intimacy with a beloved mate.

With some effort, skill, and goodwill, a loving intimacy can be preserved, or reestablished, between you and your partner. Much as the buildup of little, negative things can slowly tear the fabric of a relationship, the growing accumulation of little, positive things can reknit it together. In this chapter, we'll discuss overcoming barriers to closeness, finding time for your relationship, having good conversations, healing old hurts, and rekindling romance and a comfortable sexuality.

Of course, protecting and improving any friendship has the greatest chance of success when there's a foundation of civility, empathy, and teamwork, since it's normal to be reluctant to get close—especially physically—to someone you feel routinely let down or hurt by, or angry at.* If there's currently a good deal of arguing, we suggest both partners make a personal commitment not to fight for at least a week or two—and hopefully longer. When it starts to get heated, take a break to cool

* As we said in chapter 6, if there is threatened or actual physical abuse in your relationship, please contact a therapist or women's shelter immediately. You should not attempt to use this chapter with your partner until there is no possibility of violence between you.

off, talk about it after you've eaten or slept, or bring in a third party to help you stay calm. If you can manage even just a couple of weeks without angry conflicts, it's remarkable how much better it will feel between you. Down the road, when your relationship is stronger, you'll be able to have the normal quarrels of any couple. But now's the time for each of you to choose words carefully and be on your best behavior.

People approach their relationship from different places. Hopefully, you and your partner have preserved a reservoir of love and passion for each other and just need to carve out more time to talk or bring a little more life into your romantic relationship. But maybe you have grown emotionally distant: Even if you work well as a team, your hearts are not as connected as they once were. And for some couples, it's sad to say that their relationship is in real trouble. We'll present a range of suggestions in this chapter for this range of needs; if things are generally good between you and your partner, please don't be alarmed by the comments or options offered to couples that are in a more difficult situation.

The more strained the relationship, the more effort that's needed to turn it around—but that's also when it's hardest to bite one's tongue, or be understanding, friendly, or affectionate. How do you motivate yourself to move toward each other when you want to pull back, to give when you're aching to receive, and to respond to the other person's grievances when you feel so wronged?

It's not easy. At different times in our own relationships, we've been there, so we know how hard it can be. But certain things can really help you stay motivated to work on your marriage:

- Remember the love you once had. There was a time when you were very fond of each other: If it could happen then, it can happen again.
- Understand the reasons why you and your partner have distanced from each other (these are discussed in the next section).

Insight into them lessens their power over you and makes it easier to restore more warmth in your relationship.

- Have faith that if you make a serious and sustained effort yourself, the relationship will almost certainly get better. Imagine a scale running from zero to one hundred: Zero is no effort for the relationship, and one hundred is the absolute maximum that anyone could possibly do. In our experience, when either partner (ideally, both) consistently operates in the thirties or forties on that scale for several weeks in a row, the relationship always gets better. By two or three months, there's a *dramatic* improvement. And if they can get up into the eighties or nineties for a good deal of this time, the change in their marriage can be extraordinary. In other areas, most of us have made this much effort numerous times, such as pushing hard at work for a few months, getting through a tough semester in college, training for something athletic—or for long stretches while raising children. In those areas, people make strong efforts with hardly a thought, yet when it comes to an important relationship, suddenly it seems like an odd idea to work this hard. But why not? The stakes are greater and the chance of success just as good. A relationship is like anything else: It usually gets a lot better when you work at it.
- If your relationship has really deteriorated, you can sometimes motivate yourself to work on it by remembering that divorce is painful and difficult. Yes, there are times when things have gotten to such a state of rancor that separating is the least-bad alternative. But having read the research and seen many divorces—or, in Ricki's case, lived through one—it's a plain fact that most children suffer in a divorce, and many are injured psychologically as well. The initial breakup is stressful for both parents and children, and even when things

> settle down, there's usually a wound in the family that lasts for years: It can include more room to diverge in parenting practices, financial disruption, grappling with new partners or stepparents, and upsetting challenges in scheduling holidays. You'll probably see your children less, and when you have them, solo parenting is no picnic—one reason why single mothers tend to have worse physical and mental health than married ones. Children—and their mom and dad—do survive divorce, but the costs are such that we think it's both principled and self-interested for parents to do *everything* they can to prevent it.

As we said earlier, while it would be best if your partner went through this chapter with you, we couldn't be sure that would happen, so it's written as if only you will read it. That focus on what *you* could do, understandably, can make you feel like you have to do all the work. We feel strongly that a father should make a serious effort to nurture his partner and their relationship, and if anything, he should be the one to put more into the marriage since she is probably more depleted than he is. But meanwhile, there are two kinds of things you can do that do not depend on him: You can keep telling him what you need in your relationship, and you can try to be a better partner yourself.

Neither of these means that you are letting him off the hook, "enabling him," or putting the burden of the relationship entirely on your own shoulders. You are just doing what you can to build the intimate friendship that will nurture you—and the effort alone will make you feel strong in yourself, active instead of helpless, filled with positive energy, dignified and honorable. Your efforts will likely evoke similar steps from him over time, and if they don't, you will know in your heart—and someday if you choose, would be able to say to your children—that you did everything you could to help your relationship get better.

If things have gotten bad in a marriage, there's often a kind of no-win standoff in which he says, *I'll change if she changes,* while she says, *I'll change if he does.* The only way to break that deadlock is for someone to emphasize his or her own efforts to make the relationship better; the 80-20 principle discussed in the previous chapter applies to intimate friendship as well as to teamwork. Ideally, both partners would do so. But if he doesn't, what's your best option? Even though it's hard and it's not fair, the most direct way for you to have a better relationship is to take action on your own to improve it.

UNDERSTANDING AND OVERCOMING BLOCKS TO INTIMACY

As much as you know in your head that you should make these efforts, your heart could be pulling in a different direction. To be sure, sometimes the reasons are healthy. For example, it may be all too clear that a partner is impaired by drugs or alcohol, violent, or mentally ill—in which case you should always seek professional help. And under any circumstances, every person needs to maintain a sense of being an autonomous individual—even when you feel most connected. There are also normal differences in the desire for closeness; some of us would like to be around people all day, while others prefer and need much more time alone.

Then, besides the natural and understandable reasons you may have for not getting *too* close, there could be some reasons that aren't so good. See if any of these eight problems that can block intimacy apply to you or your partner; if one of them does, take a look at its solutions. (To avoid a numbing repetition of both personal pronouns, we focus specifically on a mother or a father in most of these problems, though every one of them could apply to either gender.)

1. It seems like there is *no time to be together.*
   Solutions: Look ahead in this chapter for practical ways to create time for the two of you. You might also consider whether busyness has become an excuse for avoiding closeness. For example, one father admitted to Rick: *I wasn't really aware of it until recently, but for a long time now, I've been quite happy to work late. It was tense when I got home, and I knew Hallie would be on me for one thing or another, so I found myself leaving the office later and later.* And a mother said: *Luna, our two-year-old, still needs me to lie down with her at night for her to go to sleep. Doug says I have to let her learn to sleep on her own, but she cries and gets really upset, so I keep doing it. But I usually fall asleep too, so we're never together at night for talking or having fun together, which frustrates him no end. The truth is, I just don't feel very interested in him right now, especially when it seems like all he wants to talk about are problems at work. He notices my mind drifting off, which hurts him and often starts an argument. So I don't mind falling asleep with Luna. It's easier this way: He can't pester me, and we don't get into a fight about me not listening to the details of some issue with his job.*

   If you have been using (perhaps unconsciously) your circumstances as a means to the end of distancing, decide if you want to continue doing this. If you don't, you could acknowledge what's been happening to a friend or your partner as a way to get it out in the open and have more conscious control. With your partner, try to talk through and resolve the issues that make you feel like distancing. For instance, in the examples above, the father could give his wife more support so that she would feel less drained and less irritable with him, and he could ask her not to criticize him the first moment he walks through the door; the mother could put a time limit on how long she'll stay with Luna (perhaps setting a quiet little bell on her phone's timer in case she falls asleep), and suggest to Doug that they talk about some of her interests as well as his.

2. You are *emotionally drained from tending to children.*
   Solutions: At the practical level, see if it's possible to get more help from others, including your partner—especially respites in the middle of long stretches of solitary childcare. Psychologically speaking, look inside to see if the boundaries between you and your children are too porous; it's one thing to be deeply empathic, and another to feel so merged that their needs or pain become your own. Try to do more of the things that give you a stronger sense of self, like a hobby you like, exercise, or meditation. When you're together with your child, pay attention to the intensity of your feelings, and try to relax and release them if they start to seem overwhelming. Also consider if you have a greater sense of responsibility for your family than is necessary and nurturing to you. If this is the case, you could talk about it with a friend, ask for more help from others, and remember the many things besides yourself—so it's not all on your shoulders—that are promoting the welfare of your family, from a child's natural development (Mother Nature is on your side!) to the support of your partner and friends.
3. Your husband is *stressed out by and preoccupied with work.*
   Solutions: When you're the one who is concerned about something, he should empathize with you, as discussed in chapter 7. And here, the most direct way to feel more connected is to start with empathy yourself, by talking about the difficulties he's facing, his concerns, and any underlying issues in his mind (e.g., competitiveness with colleagues, fear of looking bad). Then, the two of you might be able to come up with ways

he could think about or approach his job that would make it less stressful or worrisome—from psychological methods (like recalling his past successes) to more concrete ones, such as asking for administrative support in getting out quarterly reports. Finally, try to make agreements about the "mindspace" work occupies when he's with you or his children. Maybe he needs 10 minutes to shift gears when he first gets home, and then he can be fully available for his family. He could probably agree not to take business calls at night. And he should accept the general principle that it's really important for his kids and his marriage that he be emotionally present when he is home.

4. You *think he should not ask for much from you while the kids are little*, and then you'll have energy for him again.
   Solutions: While it's realistic for parents to expect less from each other in the way of intimate friendship while raising young children, it's a mistake to think you can put your partner in the deep freeze for a few years, then pop him in the microwave and expect everything to be warm and tasty between you again. During peak demand times—such as the first months after childbirth, while an infant is colicky, or when either of you is sick or flat-out exhausted—it's understandable if you have less capacity for physical or emotional connection. But in general, there's no way around a simple fact: We have to keep investing in an intimate friendship if we want to continue to have one.

We've heard moms contemptuously describe the yearnings of their partners for more attention and affection as weak, needy, or childish. But it's as wrong to view them like that as it would be for your partner to describe your own desires for connection in the same way. He is a human being with feelings, and there's a good chance he misses you in some ways. These are normal needs, and small steps on your part might make a big difference. Find out what he has in mind—both what he'd really like and the minimum that could sustain him during this time in the making of your family. It may not take that much from you to do little things for your relationship within that range. And of course, you can ask for some things from him.

5. He's *withholding attention, warmth, or affection* because of his issues with you.
Solutions: The fastest way to encourage someone to treat you better is to address his issues and treat him civilly yourself. Find out what his grievances are, sort out the reasonable wheat from the unreasonable chaff, and then do what you can about his legitimate needs. Then, if he keeps holding back, you're on a solid footing to talk with him about it.

6. You are *wary of getting hurt or disappointed*.
Solutions: Further on in this chapter, we discuss how you and your partner can work through past but lingering upsets in which you felt let down or mistreated. From now on, try to make realistic agreements that will prevent that kind of painful event from ever happening again.

Inside your own mind, you could double-check that you are not overestimating the likelihood of your partner acting in a hurtful way, the intensity of your reactions if he does, and your inability to cope with the reactions you might have. Try to become increasingly aware of any ways that thoughts, feelings, or wants from your childhood are intensifying your reactions.

Reach out to other sources of nurturance for you—like friends, spiritual practice, exercise, or art—and take in what they give you, making it a part of yourself so that your emotional reserves are more filled up and there is less impact if someone lets you down. And when he does connect with you, let it sink in, feeling the love that is actually there for you, letting yourself feel more trusting and comfortable with closeness; if the moments of lovingness between you these days are few and far between, that is all the more reason to drink deep when you can.

7. Either of you sometimes feels *overwhelmed or frightened by closeness.* While we've seen this in both women and men, let's suppose that your partner is less comfortable with emotional intimacy than you are. It may seem he doesn't care much about relationships, but in fact, the opposite could be true: Because he cares so much, because he is so affected by an intimate partner, he might feel the need to put up buffers—like how a person whose pupils are dilated needs sunglasses. Without that distancing, he might feel intruded upon, swamped, or exhausted.

   Solutions: You can talk about your sense that he wants to be emotionally close, but it seems uncomfortable for him. You can suggest that he look at his tendency to seek an optimal distance, tacking back and forth between closeness and disconnection; the closer he gets, the more he wants to distance—to the point that he wants to move closer again. He can become more aware of the methods he uses to keep you at arm's length, like falling asleep while putting children to bed or getting lost in the computer at night. He can also look at any ways his mind has found to simultaneously reach out and step back, like bickering about small things: the perfect method for staying both safely separate and just connected enough.

   Based on this self-awareness, when you're together, he can keep relaxing his body, recentering, allowing your words and presence to flow through him, all the while noticing that he is still his own person, still intact, still in charge of his own mind. He can remind himself that your experience is over there while his is over here, and that he can make any decisions later, when he's had time alone to reflect. He can let you know when he needs you to dial down the emotional intensity and give him some breathing room so that he can really hear your words and feelings. All of this can help him to feel safe enough to stay connected.

On your part, you can respond to his signals to take a step back, and learn not to take his withdrawals so personally. When you respect his need for distance, he could be more able to come closer. You can also reassure him that he needn't fear he will be overwhelmed or controlled: Maybe it was that way when he was a kid, but you're not like that, and it's not going to happen today. You and he can talk about the distance or closeness you each prefer, and then come to understandings in which you both stretch to meet the other person's needs. In particular, the two of you can take steps to get out of vicious cycles in which his distancing leads to your pursuing, which makes him distance further, and so on: Your acceptance of his need for space will interrupt the cycle, and on his side, he can give you more regular experiences of connection, making you feel more fulfilled and secure, and thus less anxious or insistent—which in turn will help him feel more comfortable with closeness.

8. It feels like *overcoming sheer inertia to be loving.* Even if you know that a touch, warm smile, quick hug, compliment, or simple *I love you* would bring you closer—it can feel so hard to make that first move. Walking past each other in the hall can feel like two ships passing in the night, trailing thoughts in the wake like *I wish she'd smile* or *Why is it so hard for him to be a little affectionate?* To be sure, there is a normal range in how much affection a person wants to express or receive; some of us are gushier than others. Still, on a typical day, how often is your mate warm and loving toward you—or you toward him? In many couples after children, the answer would be zero for each person—which raises real concerns about their relationship.

Solutions: Certainly there are times when people feel so angry, wronged, or unsafe that it would be utterly false to do something to connect; the light is red: full stop. But mostly, your feelings probably move around on a spectrum ranging from orange (you're irritated but could still find some warmth for him if you tried) through yellow (neutral, task-oriented busyness) to green (a positive attitude toward him). Anywhere along that spectrum, a person really could find a genuine fondness inside and then express it. But it takes an act of will.

We use our will many times a day, whenever our inclination is to do one thing but we ask ourselves to do another: crawl out of a warm bed to walk a crying baby, listen politely to Uncle Fred tell the same story a second time, or tidy up when it would be so nice to collapse on the sofa. Nonetheless, it's uncommon to bring one's will to a matter of the heart—but it would be so helpful. Early on in a relationship, love bubbles up unbidden, and it's natural to think that wellspring will overflow forever. Yet with the passage of time, and the usual accumulation of irritations and hurts, it's normal for love to sink underground. Consequently, over the course of a typical marriage—and especially when the relationship is troubled—the only way love will be openly expressed is if someone reaches into that well, finds some fondness, and shares it.

No doubt, this can feel hard, if not impossible, to do. But each partner probably uses his or her will every day to do even harder things. And after being willfully warm a few times, there's a good chance that love will start flowing more freely between you.

Sometimes love is close to the surface, while at other times, a person has to stretch way down for it. Either way, it is real, not fake. You honor your commitment to your family by caring enough to make an effort to offer simple gestures of fondness to your partner: Loving at will is actually twice loving.

MAKING TIME FOR YOUR RELATIONSHIP

Josie—raising two sons, ages four and eight—shrugged when Rick asked about her marriage: *We're treading water. You're busier than ever, the days blur by, and then you look up and there's your husband, and you realize that it's been weeks, literally weeks, since you've done anything fun or happy together. When we do get some time, it's great and there's a little glow in our relationship that lasts a couple days. We keep saying we have to do that more often. But it's really hard.*

Yes, time apart can contain warm thoughts of each other, and grinding out tasks side by side could have a nice sense of camaraderie. But that is just not enough to recharge anyone's relationship over the long haul, particularly while it's being challenged by each partner's stress and weariness, and by conflicts related to raising a family. You need time together that feeds your relationship. The question is *how*—amid the daily rush, the bills, the dishes—and here are some suggestions.

Make it important. When people make a personal commitment to set aside more time for their relationship, they usually find some ways to do so. But without that resolve, the world, the kids, the job will grab your time and suck it up and there'll be little or nothing left for your marriage. For a motivating dose of reality, you could track (casually or carefully) the minutes each week that are actually spent talking with warmth and caring, being physically affectionate, or having fun together. With your partner, try to discuss these facts—framed as a "we" problem, not "me against you"—and say how each of you would like things to be from now on.

Do tasks together. Understandably, parents often divide their tasks in order to conquer them: Dad's in the kitchen doing dishes while Mom's giving Junior a bath. But then there's zero opportunity for closeness. Instead, try to do more tasks jointly. For example, when you're both cleaning up after dinner or bathing a child, it's easier and more fun. Additionally, look for chances to connect even while you're getting things done, like comfortably touching shoulders at the sink, shared glances of amusement at a child's play with a stuffed animal, rubbing a partner's foot as he or she reads a story, friendly conversation in the car while running errands, holding hands as you walk your child into day care, and so on.

Create family fun. You can also do more family activities that are fun and connecting for Mom and Dad, not just the kids, such as roughhousing together, making music, hide and seek, board and card games, building something, arts and crafts, making cookies, or planting flowers.

Make time for pillow talk. Arranging to go to bed at the same time gives you more private moments for talking and snuggling, but that's hard for many parents. For example, sleep is at such a premium for a nursing mother that she often goes to bed before the father does. And Rick has listened to numerous couples quarrel bitterly about one person insisting on staying up after their partner has gone to bed in order to read or watch a movie, since *That's the only time I get to myself.* Yet the difference in bedtimes is usually small enough—an hour or so at most—that it's easy to bridge with a gracious compromise. You could split the difference: If he's the night owl, he might come to bed a half hour sooner while you stay up for half an hour. Or maybe he could get the kids going in the morning, giving you more time to sleep so you can go to bed later with him. Or he might come to bed with you, talk and cuddle for a while, and then go back out to another room.

Establish daily routines. Try to build time for just the two of you into the normal rhythm of your day. Tell the kids to leave you alone—perhaps after setting them up with an activity—and make the rule stick; soon enough, almost any child past two will come to respect it. Some couples have a glass of wine or cup of tea together when they're both home from work. You could arrange for the kids to eat early so you can have a peaceful dinner with each other. Firm bedtimes will give you time to yourselves in the evening. Or pay an older child to play with your younger ones for a few hours over the weekend while you hang out together in another part of your home; a friendly ten-year-old is a preschooler's dream playmate.

Schedule regular date nights. By the time most infants are six months old (and for some, it's sooner), they can handle their parents going off for an hour or so in the evening. At this point, try to schedule a "date night" at least once a month, and maybe even weekly. The first time or two, let yourself be as careful or nervous as you like: Call home every 15 minutes, talk about the kids the whole time at dinner, leave the movie early because you can't stand being away from your baby, whatever—we've been there. But soon it will feel very natural, and the kids will see it as simply part of the weekly routine. Some couples swap babysitting with each other, so you get your date night this week and they have theirs the next one. Babysitting co-ops are a more elaborate version of this basic idea; you could ask around to see if there is a good one in your area—or maybe start one yourself.

Refresh your relationship. But now that you're together, sometimes it's been so long that you're not quite sure what to do or how to be! As one mom put it: *We went out for the first time after Luis was born, ordered dinner, and then just kind of stared at each other. Finally, we both started laughing, it was so silly and awkward. We had been so busy for months with the baby that we had sort of forgotten how to be together as just us. It felt strange, shy.* For ideas—plus rekindling fond memories—you could talk about what you liked doing together when you first started dating, or at any time pre-kids. It's also worth thinking about new activities that would bring fresh interest and energy to your relationship. How about taking turns picking something new to do each month? Try to share the load of orchestrating these activities instead of letting it fall on one person to make all the arrangements.

Let good moments last. Even when both people want things to be good between them, it's striking how hard it can be to let the nice moments last. Every one of the barriers to intimacy discussed in the previous section can get in the way. For example, a part of you may not want to open into strong feelings of liking or love. Perhaps you fear this would imply that your past complaints were not valid. Maybe it would feel too vulnerable to open up to good feelings with your partner and risk being hurt again. So then you might not see opportunities to build a nice interaction, or do something that spoils the moment and puts you at odds with each other again.

Instead, try to remember all the reasons—from the long overdue healing of your heart to the benefits for your children—for letting warm feelings linger between you. Take the moment for what it is. These minutes together are like beads on your life's necklace: Will they be pearls, or something plain or painful? You can help them be good by stretching yourself to be present when you feel far away, open rather than guarded. Try to find the goodness and vulnerability in him that naturally evokes warmth and caring in you. When he offers something positive, try to build on it rather than letting it hit the ground with a thud. Protecting these moments makes a sanctuary for your love, giving it room to live—and grow.

ASKING THREE QUESTIONS A DAY

Many couples would say that talking together was once the best part of their relationship. One mother told Rick: *He always made me laugh. When we started dating, sometimes we'd talk on the phone for three hours. It was just stuff: office weirdness, where to go skiing, some hassle we'd had. But I could hear him breathing; he felt so close to me. I really miss that. We still talk, but never for very long, and it's usually very practical: the kids, the house, info, problems. I'd say we still have a strong marriage, and I'm grateful for that. Yet it's strange: I miss him even though I see him every day.*

Yet now, real conversation—that goes beyond *How was it with Alan today?* Or *I called the guy about the insurance*—gets pushed to the side by childcare, housework, and the pressures of making a living: Who's got time to talk anymore?! So when we do, it's much more about exchanging information, driving toward decisions, and maybe arguing. It's a pity, since conversation is a crucial way to stay connected, especially for many women—and particularly for one who's spent most of her day in the company of children.

So consider asking each other at least three questions a day. Questions about each other, not the bills, the dry cleaning, or the company picnic. Questions that do not carry implicit criticism or advice. Questions that contain real interest, that reach out, like: *What do you think about that? How did it make you feel? What would you really like?* Questions that make you feel more connected when you're done than when you started.

Some of the time, you'll be talking about your reactions to everyday matters such as little events of the day. It's also important to understand the hopes and dreams of each other, with questions like these: *When you were a kid, what did you want to be when you grew up? Are you generally satisfied with your life, or do you feel something important is missing? If you suddenly had three extra hours each day, what would you do with them?*

No matter the topic, though, try to stay out of an argument when you're in "asking three questions" mode. In particular, these conversations may not be the best time to get into "our relationship." For some, broaching that subject comes from an effort to connect, but for others, it could seem to contain a built-in criticism. If that topic brings you closer, fine, but if not, see if you can save it for another occasion.

There's a place for graciousness, for bringing your attention to something that may not be your preference in the moment. A place for shifting gears inside your mind and letting yourself be drawn into a topic—and more importantly—into a sense of relationship with your partner. Both of you could cultivate a quality of being fully present, relaxed, and open to this moment together. It helps to notice the kinds of mental chatter that take you out of the moment, and take fewer rides on those trains of thought.

HEALING BRUISES TO YOUR RELATIONSHIP

Relationships require repairs. Occasional misunderstandings, disappointments, and resentments are the rule, not the exception. Many of these fade with time and good experiences together. But some may linger, darkening the mood of a relationship, leading partners to shrink it to a size that feels safe, and adding dynamite to quarrels over little things. By healing old wounds, you and your partner will feel more trusting and loving. You'll like each other more, your relationship will be stronger when the next challenge comes—and there won't be any explosives gathering dust in a corner of the living room.

Common Relationship Issues Between Parents

Many couples face one or more of these issues related to having a family:

- They had serious disagreements about having children in the first place.
- They had to deal with upsetting and expensive fertility procedures in order to conceive their child.
- She felt he distanced during her pregnancy, or he wasn't understanding when she had a miscarriage; or during childbirth, he wasn't emotionally present or supportive.
- He felt she started losing interest in him during her pregnancy, and then especially since their baby was born.
- She felt he let her down in the most important undertaking of her life.
- They had widely different ideas about how to raise their children.
- Someone said or did something terrible during a fight.
- He felt she has indulged herself in the private pleasures of being a mother and hasn't pulled her weight in bringing money into the family.
- She felt pressured by him to go to work when she wanted to stay home, or to stay home when she wanted to go to work.
- He felt stung by her micromanagement of his parenting, her obvious view of him as a kind of clueless Fred Flintstone.
- She's sick and tired of him criticizing the housework—especially when he does so little himself.

- She stopped being interested in him sexually.
- He felt abandoned by her, emotionally and romantically, once children arrived.
- Someone had an affair.

Out with the Old

Over the years, we've found certain questions to be helpful in healing hurts and getting a relationship back on track. Besides considering them privately, you can discuss them with each other, either informally or by setting aside specific times. When you do talk, try to keep in mind the methods covered in the two previous chapters, including civility, empathy, and sharing your own experience without blame or defensiveness. It could work best if one person at a time talks about a question completely (or several questions in a row), before the other person does—or you may prefer to go back and forth within a question in a less structured way. You can also explore the questions in any order that suits you. Take your time with them: They cover a lot of ground, and some may be so loaded that you have to approach them gently. If you can talk productively on your own, great. But if not, it could help to have a third person present, like a clergy member, a trusted friend or relative, or a therapist.

Here are the questions, which each partner could answer:

1. What were your original hopes and dreams for your relationship, before children? What did you want to give? What did you hope you would receive?
2. What did you imagine life with children would be like? What did you anticipate would be the effects of children on your relationship?

3. What have been the *actual* effects of children on your relationship? Such as on your energy level, finances, time, romance, sexuality, emotional intimacy, or conflicts?
4. What has made things go badly between you? (No blame, just the facts; don't refight those quarrels . . .) To be honest, how have you brought out qualities in your mate that bother you? (Like how one person's stonewalling of criticism makes the other person more insistent.)
5. How have you suffered in your relationship? And—painful question—how have you made your partner suffer? Related to each other, how have you each felt anger? Hurt? Shame? Loss? Fear? Sadness? What could you have compassion for, both in yourself and in your partner?
6. How might you have misunderstood some of your partner's motives or feelings? How might you have interpreted his or her actions in an unnecessarily negative way? How might your childhood have affected, intensified, or distorted your reactions to your partner? Your life experiences prior to marriage? Your growing sensitization to certain issues with your partner?
7. What have you tried to do to make your relationship better? What has worked well when you stuck with it?
8. What has kept you from sticking with the things that work for your relationship—both external circumstances and internal thoughts, attitudes, or feelings? For example, how have other parts of your daily life gotten to be a higher priority than caring for your relationship? What has felt scary to you about being vulnerable, or giving your partner a fresh chance? What might be the hidden rewards to you of the problems in your relationship—such as proving that he's done you wrong, or making you feel justified (and not a bad person) in seeking a divorce?

9. What feels correct and wise to take more responsibility for in your relationship? To apologize for? To ask forgiveness for?
10. Stated cleanly, without blame or rancor, what would you like to request from your partner? What would you like your partner to take more responsibility for? Apologize for? Do differently in the future?
11. What could you do differently to make your relationship better—both outward behaviors and internal actions within your own mind? What forgiveness and letting go could you extend to your partner? How could you help each other stay on track? How could you help yourself?

As a speaker, try to focus on communicating for yourself, not on any response you might want from your partner. Be clear on your purpose: to express whatever will help to release this upset, getting it out of your nervous system and out of your relationship—that's your priority, ahead of being right, winning the point, or paying him back. As you share your experience, try to sense that it's leaving your body and no longer troubling your mind. Notice the depth of your partner's listening and his sincere attempts to understand and clean up the mess. Let in his compassion, his regrets and remorse, and his commitment to act differently in the future. As the speaker, see if you can let go of the upset, and move on.

When you're the listener, remember that you have an opportunity here to release this upset from your relationship. Help your partner get everything out in the open, especially whatever is hard to say. Try to get down to the bottom of his upset; you want to pull the tip of the root so that it doesn't grow back. Say back what you understand—particularly the deeper feelings, wants, or bruises—so your partner knows you got it. Try to acknowledge as much validity as possible in his views. Take as much responsibility as you authentically can for your part of the upset. State your regrets or remorse for everything you can. Say what you would have done differently in the past if you had only known better, and what you will do differently from this point forward. As the listener, see if you can let go of the upset, and move on.

In with the New

It is very important to keep any agreements you made with each other in these conversations. When you've been let down in the past, and then warily extend the open hand of trust one more time, there's a particularly bitter slump of disappointment if it happens again. Also, the growing closeness between you might stir up fears of vulnerability and hurt, so it is common for couples to slip into an argument in order to return to a familiar sense of distance. You could discuss some of the ways this might happen, and how you could prevent it.

Further, as you look to the future, how will you cultivate even more love for each other? Healing upsets is like pulling weeds. But it's not growing flowers. A couple can get to a place where neither person is really mad at the other one, but there is a numbness or exhaustion in the relationship. Maybe you wonder: *Will I ever really love him again? Will I even like him again? Will he be loving with me?* Sometimes the heart has become so stony that it seems nothing green will ever grow there again. But when just a little effort is sustained, we've seen a kind of miracle happen many times: pockets of fondness and caring beginning to emerge, fragile at first, then spreading and getting sturdier, love taking hold, softening a once-hardened heart.

It feels mainly like love happens *to* us, but we can also consciously plant its seeds within ourselves, protect them, and help them grow. If you think about yourself—and these points apply just as much to your partner—the seeds of a lasting love include:

- A general attitude of being compassionate and kind toward everyone—including your partner
- A sense of the being behind his eyes, seen through the filters—perhaps a little overgrown these days—of his personality
- Allowing warmth, liking, and love to come forward within you—not putting a lid on these to prove a point or pay him back
- Actions that are friendly, caring, interested, loving—even when they are not your first thought in the moment, but are still authentic—which evoke those real feelings within you
- Doing things together that naturally lead to warm feelings, like recalling good times together
- Honoring him as your co-parent, joined in the difficult, wondrous undertaking of raising a family

SEX AFTER CHILDREN

Ah, sex. After children come along, it becomes an issue for many couples. There is little time or opportunity—and often not much interest in one or both partners. But based on a foundation of teamwork, emotional safety, friendship, and nonsexual affection, romance and sweet lovemaking can help keep a marriage healthy, or help reknit one that's unraveling.

> *Helpful husbands are an aphrodisiac for their wives.*
>
> A mother

First, some clarifications. We don't mean sex when it's uncomfortable during pregnancy or for some months after childbirth. We don't mean sex on demand, sex that might lead to an unwanted pregnancy, or sex with someone you really don't like very much right now. But when the dust settles some months after a baby is born, we suggest making an effort to preserve a romantic and erotic dimension in your marriage, living together as lovers as well as friends and co-parents.

If you and your partner are both happy with your sex life, that's great. But difficulties related to sex are not uncommon, as you can see in these blunt comments from one woman on a survey Rick handed out at a mothers' club: *We've got one child, 8 months old. I work full-time, commute 45 minutes to work each way, have two dogs to walk daily, and handle 100 percent of the housework. My husband works for a high-tech company, with lots of pressure, a long commute and long work day, and he also has to get up early to check emails. He'd like to make love once a week, but I'd choose about once every two months, so we do it about once a month. Every night, we are both exhausted. When he complains that I'm not interested, I try to reassure him that I'm just tired. Weirdly enough, if I walk the dogs for an extra long period, he thinks I must be having an affair! Tell me, is there* any *mom with little kids out there with the energy for* two *men?!*

Like many couples, you might be dealing with one of these issues:

- One partner—often the man, but not always—is more interested in sex than the other one.
- Neither of you is very interested in sex per se, but a spark is definitely missing in your relationship.
- Practical problems are getting in the way of your love life, such as no good times, kids crying right when you get started, awkward to shift from mommy/daddy mode to lover mode, etc.

The first two of these are about *wants*, while the last one is about *arrangements*. Let's start with the more fundamental issue—sexual desire—and then tackle the normal difficulties that complicate a romantic, erotic relationship after children.

But I Don't Want To

At this point, it is possible that somewhere in your mind a voice is saying something like: *That's all well and good. But what if I just don't want to?*

Of course, you absolutely don't have to. We've known some long and happy marriages in which both people were content with little or no sex. But that's pretty rare. The lack of an erotic aspect means that there is less to bring—and keep—the couple together. It may indicate deeper issues that need attention. And it creates conflicts if one partner wishes for more erotic contact than the other one does.

Besides leaving things as they are, you and your mate have four options if there's a disparity of desire:

- You both can accept your differences.
- The one who wants more becomes satisfied with less.
- The one who wants less kindles the desire for more.
- You both can make gracious accommodations.

Many couples weave their way through a combination of these, emphasizing one more than another at different times. We've tried each one and can vouch for them. But above all, whatever you do has to feel like it's your own decision, not forced upon you in any way—and this is especially true if you've experienced sexual abuse or assault, or grew up in an oversexualized atmosphere. Sex is highly charged, and some people can be very persuasive—or even threatening or intimidating—to get what they want. It's alright for one partner to make their case or express their feelings. Then they need to step back enough for you to make your own choices. Let's look closely at what you might be choosing.

Will Change Diapers for Sex: Accepting Your Differences

Ironically, coming together about sex starts with acknowledging the ways in which you are apart. Sex is one of those aspects of life in which there is enormous natural variation in desire and preferred practices. One source of this variety is, obviously, gender: In most straight couples—and especially those with children—the man has a greater sex drive. (If it's not like that in your relationship, see the box, and you can apply much of the rest of this chapter by simply switching the genders.) The difference in natural interest is often a source of friction, as you can see in this imaginary, plainspoken dialogue, a condensed version of what we've heard from many mothers and fathers:

She says: *For starters, you need to understand that my body was already overtouched long before you came near me, I'm tired most of the time, and the last thing I'm looking forward to when I finally get to bed is an aerobic activity. It's not personal if I'd rather go to sleep. The truth is, I don't feel sexual a lot of the time—and I'm not just neutral about it: At those times, deep in my brain, I want to* not *be sexual. This is really how most mothers are. Ask a hundred women with little kids where they'd put sex on a list of ten pleasant ways to spend a half hour—including taking a long bath, reading a magazine, or chatting with a friend—and most of them would put it near the bottom or even off the list altogether. I know your list would be different, that sex would be at or near the top. That's normal for you. But my list is normal for me.*

Once we get past that generic lack of initial interest, yes, I still enjoy sex with you. But it has to be based on something. I need to feel that you care about me, the person, much more than you lust after the body I inhabit. Since many women have been treated like a sexual object, you can understand why I need your leading communication to be one of cherishing and respect. And it's got to be real, not a box you're trying to check off so you can get to what you want. I can't have sex in order to connect; I need to feel connected in order to have sex.

Foreplay starts in the morning, when you support me in the care of our children, pulling your weight, showing through your deeds that you value what I value. To be blunt, I need to feel that we're joined in raising a family in order to be interested in joining my body with yours in bed. And foreplay continues throughout the day in how we talk with and treat each other. There's a switch inside me (and most women, I bet) that's set firmly to "off" whenever it doesn't feel good and safe between us. I need to have made up with you before I can start making out.

And there'll be many times when you're doing everything right, and I still won't want sex. It could be the kids crying, which is a total turnoff. Maybe I'm worn out, or my body feels funny. Whatever it is, it's not about you. You really shouldn't take it personally. And when you do get mad at me about not having sex, I become even less interested.

When He's Less Interested in Sex Than You Are

A man could have less desire for sex than his partner does for a variety of reasons. Some have nothing to do with being a father, such as naturally low libido that preceded children, physical shyness, concerns about performance, or a partner who has a naturally higher interest in sex than he does. Parenthood-related reasons could include upsets with his partner about raising a family, not feeling attracted to her physically after her body has changed due to having children, seeing her as a motherly figure rather than an erotic partner, or being unwilling to approach her after being repeatedly rejected.

Some mothers are content with the situation, because they have little interest in sex themselves, and a partner's lack of interest takes the pressure off them. Others feel resigned, although the status quo is not their preference and they're troubled about the long-term implications for the marriage. And some women are hurt and frustrated.

If you wish your partner were more interested in sex, see if you can talk with him openly about it. Find out the reasons for his lack of interest, perhaps using the ones given above as a starting point. If he has no desire for sex at all (typically indicated by never or rarely masturbating), that often suggests depression, sexual dysfunction, or a medical problem. He should talk with a therapist or physician; your support will be a key element in things getting better in this aspect of your relationship. If he isn't interested in sex with *you*, it's prudent to make sure he's not having an affair or seeing a sex worker. Once you've eliminated these unlikely possibilities, find out if there is anything you could do differently, such as resolve an upset between you, reassure him in some way, give him longer foreplay (which men need as they grow older), adjust to his preferred times to make love, or perhaps try some new things in bed. But none of that means doing anything that feels emotionally wrong or degrading. And in the end, you can only do so much, and the ultimate source of the solution(s) to his sexual issues will have to be him.

He says: *I'm a normal man, and I think sex is one of the major good things in life. My attraction to you hasn't changed just because we've had children. But none of that means I don't also see you as a whole person, or don't care about your mind and soul. I want to have sex with you* because *I love you. It's a physical expression of my love, one that's fun, sweet, and instantly connecting.*

That's why it hurts so much when you act like I'm some sort of jerk if I reach out to you sexually. When I was a boy, I had my share of painful moments of feeling rejected, and I don't need any more of those.

Occasionally, I want to be seen and wanted as a lover, not just a breadwinner or someone who can give a child a bath. I can totally understand if intercourse is physically uncomfortable for you, but if that's not an issue, I hope we can make love regularly. That sense of sex as a normal part of our relationship takes away any hurt if you're not interested tonight, since there's a good chance we'll make love pretty soon.

The real hurt for me isn't about sex per se. It's that you just don't seem to care very much about me.

I totally love our children. And I love it when we're all together. But I also want to have a relationship with you that's about just you and me. I married you because I love you, I cherish you, and I want to be with you. So when I try to draw you into relationship with me, whether it's just us talking or we're in bed and the door's locked, it is not in order to drive a wedge between you and our children. I don't want you to give them less, I just want you to carve out a little more space in your mind and in your day for me. It won't take much. How long does it really take to let me know you still like me, give me a kiss, or make love?

In the fictional-but-pretty-common dialogue above, it's like she's waltzing while he wants to tango. In some couples, there's a good-humored acceptance of these differences that makes it possible to work around them: They create a foundation of teamwork and intimacy that doesn't involve sex, he respects her need for a loving warm-up, she makes room in her heart for regular lovemaking—and they find ways to keep dancing together, mainly a gentle waltz, and occasionally a hot tango. But in other couples, there is less understanding and acceptance—and more conflict.

I'm right and you're wrong. One or both partners could think that their own way is what's natural and right, and that the other person needs fixing. We've done this ourselves, in our own relationships, and it's always led to conflict and pain. Instead, each parent should try to see the sexual nature of his or her partner in a neutral, open-minded way.

From your side of the bed, try to notice any lurking contempt for male sexuality—such as *Men think mostly with their little head instead of their big one*—or any exaggeration of his behavior; as a mother once said to Ricki: *All he ever thinks about is rubbing up against me. It's disgusting.* Try to find compassion for his feelings about reaching out and being routinely turned down, his sense of being unwanted, his hurt that this need of his doesn't seem to matter much in the relationship.

From his side, he can understand that having children literally alters the hormonal chemistry of your body. It is normal for estrogen to be lower than usual for several months after childbirth (longer if you continue to nurse), and estrogen helps make women receptive to sexual advances. Both stress and nursing increase production of prolactin, a serious lust-buster. He can recognize that it makes biological sense for mothers to evolve internal brakes that stop them from conceiving one child right after the other.

Even without factoring in the effects of children, he can understand that the results of sex—pregnancy and 20-plus years of motherhood—and therefore sex itself have been enormously more consequential for females than males throughout history. As a result, a woman may need more conditions to be met for making love than a man does: more stability and safety in the relationship, more vitality in her body, more confidence that he's going to love and support her in the years to come.

He can have compassion for you if you feel torn between your wish to make him happy and the plain truth that you'd rather not have sex right now. He can see that it's not about him that you're tired after a long day with a job and kids, that it's a lot of work to shift gears from mommy mode to lover mode, and that much of the time, you just don't want to want sex. He can respect your right not to want something he wants.

We need to understand each other. Perhaps you and your partner can talk frankly about your sexual natures at this time. One way would be to read the statements of the fictional mother and father and say what fits for each of you. You might even write a letter to each other that says what you understand about the other person and sex, what you'd like to have understood about you, and what you'd like to have happen in the future.

Less formally, both of you could just talk freely about sex, your likes and dislikes, your similarities and differences. You might agree to a truce in which you accept your differences and put them on hold for a while, perhaps to get through an especially demanding time. Alternatively, on a foundation of accepting each other, you could explore the following options.

Becoming Satisfied with Less

Much as a mother might take steps to encourage more sexual interest within herself (see the next section), a father could just as well take action to lower his desire for sex.

Cultivate compassion and wisdom. Based on compassion, not guilt, he can let himself feel how his sexual interest may be a kind of burden on his wife, and on the relationship. He might consider the chain reaction of effects, perhaps, on his children, his wife, and himself, and ask: *Are the rewards worth the price?* Through wisdom, seeing the greatest good for the greatest number, there could be a natural relinquishing of desire.

Sublimate sex. Like people have done throughout history, he could sublimate sexual passion into other activities. He might return to an old hobby or find a new one. Or get into some sport, go fishing more often, make some art, or climb a mountain.

Find other ways to be connected or intense. Sexuality has many elements, some of which are not sexual per se, such as closeness, intensity, affection, feeling wanted or appreciated, and physical pleasure. He could satisfy these in other ways than sex, both within and outside your relationship. For instance, he and you could make a special effort to spend more time touching or in a state of loving closeness. He could deepen his friendships with other men, finding in their company some of the companionship he has sought through sex with you. He might explore activities that provide a different kind of intensity, like rock climbing, bicycle racing, or playing music—especially vital for a man who feels a strong pull toward the wild and has used sex in part as an outlet or safety valve.

Kindling a Desire for More

Many factors—some situational and others more fundamental—affect sexual desire. In the next section, we'll look at practical ways to maintain a sexual relationship in the everyday situations of raising a family. But here, let's consider the foundations of a mother's sexuality. There are numerous ways to increase a person's authentic interest in sexual relations; you could try one (or more) of them and see if it works for you. With a little effort, we usually can genuinely want one thing less, or truly want something else more. The mind is amazingly plastic, and most of us never make a sustained push to nudge it in one direction or another. We usually don't know what is really possible within the mind until we give it a try. Of course, these are simply options, and whether you explore them is a very personal choice that is entirely up to you.

Establish a loving intimacy. When there is anything awry in the relationship, sex for most women goes right out the window. If that's part of the problem, this chapter and the two before it contain many ways to develop a warmer, closer sense of connection.

Nurture your health. Any drop in physical health will usually reduce sex drive, which is one more reason to get a thorough assessment, and to take good care of your body (see chapters 4 and 5).

Look into your hormones. You could talk with your gynecologist and assess the hormones that might be affecting your sexuality. Then there's the tough question: Do you intervene or not? Taking hormones is a tricky business for any woman, but especially for a mother. Low doses of supplemental testosterone, estrogen, progesterone, or DHEA may bring back some erotic interest. But we've also seen this backfire, producing side effects like irritability, aggressiveness, and insomnia, while disturbing a hormonal equilibrium that was already fragile in a depleted mother. If you and your doctor decide to try these approaches, it's wise to be cautious and go slowly.

Consider your medicines. Certain drugs, such as antidepressants or blood pressure medications, can lower libido altogether, not just make it hard to climax. You should discuss these possibilities with your doctor and consider other options. Nonpharmacological interventions for depressed mood—including therapy, social support, or exercise—might help your sex life. Some antidepressants have fewer sexual side effects, and the natural antidepressants Saint-John's-wort and 5-hydroxytryptophan (see chapter 5) usually do not affect sexuality. If you stick with the original medication, your doctor might suggest lowering the dose, or taking a "drug holiday" (e.g., skipping the antidepressant Friday and Saturday, and making love Sunday morning).

Get exercise. Exercise boosts energy in general and may increase sexual interest.

Care for postpartum depression. Much like depression in general, postpartum depression (PPD) usually reduces or eliminates one's interest in sex. PPD calls for treatment as a whole, not focused on the symptom of low libido. With time and good care, an interest in sex should return if PPD is the main source of your lack of desire.

Try to lift your mood. A glum mood can rob you of any interest in sex. If you've been feeling blue, "flat," or dispirited, or you've lost interest in activities that you once enjoyed, take a look at chapter 3, and perhaps talk to a therapist.

High levels of anxiety can have much the same effect as low mood. If that's a problem for you, also take a look at chapter 3, and think about contacting a therapist.

Consider your upbringing. In certain home environments or cultures, girls and women are taught that sex is somehow embarrassing, even dirty—so they are not supposed to seek or enjoy it. Or there may have been early experiences of being punished or shamed for sexual activities. As a result, your erotic desire may have become inhibited.

If you have an inkling that this might apply to you, you could use the techniques in chapters 2 and 3, read books written by women with similar upbringings, talk about it with a close friend, or see a therapist. If a person chooses not to be sexual, that is her absolute right, but the option itself may have been taken away from you. You have a right to reclaim it and then decide yourself how you will express your sexuality.

Enjoy being excited in general. Sex is about excitement, but some girls grow up with little brakes inside about being energetic, intense, spontaneous, carried away, or loud. In nonsexual situations, you could occasionally turn up the dial to a higher setting and see how that feels. You might detect a fear inside of scolding or embarrassment, and if you do, you can work with and release that fear, using methods we've previously explored. The point is to make sure that the normal human capacity for excitement is open inside you, and then you can make your own choices about what you'll do with it.

Remember previous enjoyable intimate experiences. Many people sometimes feel an initial lack of interest in sex, but after some minutes of affectionate contact, they become more interested. You could remember this the next time your partner expresses his own interest.

Turn on your mind. You could deliberately put your attention on romantic or sexual stimuli as a way to prime the pump of desire. For example, a client of Jan's told her: *I've been reading romance novels lately, and they've got me more interested in, well, romance. They're fun to read, and I like the effects.* There is a range of possibilities, starting with warm thoughts about your husband or an image of him looking particularly handsome. You could imagine teasing or dating him, or perhaps recall a time in your life when you felt especially flirtatious.

Get to know the lover within you. What is your sense of yourself as (at least sometimes) a sexual being? What is she like, this lover within you? If you were to imagine a conversation with her, what would she say, and how would she ask you to help her? When alone sometime, you might pretend to walk around your bedroom like her, and notice any differences from the ways you normally move. Can you make more room for her in your life?

Making Accommodations for Each Other

Disparities in desire often become so polarized that they look more extreme than they actually are. It's like you feel 80 feet apart and you've got a 4-foot board for a bridge—but in fact, you're only 8 feet apart, and if you each took just one step forward, it would be simple to span the gap.

We've seen many couples make accommodations for each other in the erotic arena. Honestly, we've done it ourselves. The couple comes to an understanding that works for each person, typically along these lines:

- ✦ Maintaining a foundation of teamwork and intimacy—as well as a sense of perspective about sex, making it neither a bigger nor smaller issue than it really ought to be

- The father making an effort to respect a mother's need to have surplus energy to even contemplate sex, a loving and affectionate foundation, and the right to say no without it becoming an upset
- The mother making an effort to feel comfortable with regular lovemaking
- Both having a shared understanding about how often they will, in fact, have sex

Regarding the big question—How Often Are We Going to Do It? (which usually means someone has an orgasm, though not necessarily through intercourse)—there are several approaches:

- Never or rarely, right now: Appropriate at some point during pregnancy or the first months after childbirth; usually not healthy for a long-term relationship
- Once a month: Common during pregnancy or the first year or so after childbirth; will not satisfy most men—nor many women—over the long run
- Two or three times a month: Perhaps most common for parents of young children
- Once or twice a week: Could be a father's preferred frequency of sex (though many men wouldn't mind more). Could be a stretch for a mother, but if you can find your way to being comfortable with this amount, there would be a nice glow in your relationship, and sex would disappear as an issue
- His week/her week: In the common situation in which he is more interested than she is, she'd agree to a receptivity during his week unless something occurs such as a cold or her period, and he'd follow her lead and accept a "no" during her week; perhaps not an option for a mother with a young baby, but

worth considering for mothers of older children or to break logjams around sex

We have known some couples that made effective agreements about sex without ever getting explicit. If that approach works for you, great, but if not, then you will probably need to be more plainspoken. Even if it's awkward, it usually helps to be pretty specific about what you want from each other, both outward behaviors *(please do this, never do that)* and internal attitudes. Try to listen to each other without arguing. This information is pure gold: Each of you is saying what you need in order to give your partner what he or she wants.

But even more than skillfully working out the details, it helps to be gracious and willful when you try this option of making accommodations with each other. For example, there might be a rather loose analogy between having conversations and having sex. For some people, giving themselves over to a complex and potentially emotional conversation with their partner is not their most preferred way to spend the next half hour, no matter how much they cherish that person and are committed to their relationship. But they could remind themselves that intimate conversation is good for their relationship and family, and that they usually feel better afterward. So they bring both graciousness and will to the encounter. They might remember past conversations that felt good and shift mentally from task mode to talk mode. In sum, they find and then feed a genuine motivation inside for talking. In the beginning, they may not be into the conversation, but pretty soon they get engaged and start bringing their own interests into it. Afterward, they notice good feelings inside and appreciate the effects of the conversation in their relationship, and are usually glad they took the time for it.

On the other hand, for some people, making love is not their own most preferred way to spend the next half hour, no matter how much they cherish their partner and are committed to their relationship. And there could be an even more visceral reluctance to engage in sex than to have a conversation. Still, they could remember the good reasons for making an accommodation, and bring graciousness and will to it. If there is a fair chance that sex may be a possibility later in the day, they might think a bit about some things that would make it appealing, such as warm feelings for the partner or good memories of their previous romantic experiences. At the beginning it might take a little deliberate effort to bring attention to it and to focus on what is enjoyable. And then gradually the body and mind could become more naturally engaged. Afterward, they could notice the good feelings in the relationship and be glad they were together in this way.

In both conversation and sex, there is a middle place between being effortlessly interested and absolutely opposed. We would never suggest making love if it would be painful, unsafe, abusive, or degrading. But finding a genuine willingness and comfort within yourself to spend a small amount of time—usually less than an hour each week—engaged intimately in a way that ends up feeling good for you, helps your partner feel loved, and bonds you together could be a nice way to nurture your intimate friendship.

Making Room for Two When Baby Makes Three

Now comes the logistical part. Sex was pretty simple before the baby came along: You were both interested, when and where were easy to figure out, and there were no interruptions. But now, making love seems to require a perfect configuration of children finally sleeping, no irritating interactions with kids (or each other) in the last few hours, somehow there's still some energy in your bones, the gods are smiling—and no one wakes up in the next room. These days, maintaining a spark of passion in your relationship—and igniting a fire when the time is right—takes more conscious attention than ever before.

Nonsexual affection. One of the members of a mothers' club made this interesting comment when Jan and Rick gave a talk there: *When we were first married, we touched each other all the time. At family events, people would even kid us about it. But now, I feel pretty touched-out from the kids, and it hardly occurs to me to touch him. Plus he'll think it means I want sex, and I don't, at least not then, and it would be awkward to say no, so that's another reason. And he mainly touches me when he wants sex. Which I don't like. But because about the only time we touch is when we're making love, touch has gotten equated with sex.* When she was done speaking, a dozen other women chimed in about similar situations, and we all came up with these suggestions:

- **Talk about touching:** Talk with each other about the sort of touching and affection you used to enjoy; just remembering the good feelings will get you moving in the right direction. You could also talk about how affection was expressed in the home or culture you grew up in, and how that might have put an unnecessary lid on what you're comfortable with today.
- **Ask for what you want:** Ask specifically for what you'd like, such as a kiss when you come home from work. You may think it's obvious, but your partner may have a totally different idea of what you want.
- **Let touching last:** Allow the times of touching to last longer; for example, instead of a quick pat on the back, let the hand linger. Notice any feelings that prompt you to withdraw a touch sooner than you really need to, like a discomfort with closeness or a fear that your touch will be misinterpreted.
- **Display affection in front of the kids:** Feel free to touch each other around the kids: a hand on the leg, a visible cuddle in

bed. It's not appropriate for them to witness a major make-out session—let alone anything more sexual—but it's completely fine for them to see a warm and extended hug, even if they do try to worm between you and yell, "Gross!"

- **Reach out yourself:** Besides asking him to be more affectionate, you could start touching him more on your own: on the arm, little massages, back scratches—whatever he likes. Yes, it's more giving when you may feel pretty gived-out, but try it and see what happens. Usually, it will give you a nice feeling, and he'll become more affectionate with you.
- **Experiment with affection:** Try a simple experiment, for 5 to 20 minutes each, in which you take turns being the giver and the receiver. As the giver, his job is to touch you in exactly the ways you like (though erogenous zones are off-limits), and your job is let him know when it feels good and when you'd like something different. Then you switch roles. Besides learning about the other person's preferences, you could become aware of any ways that it's hard to tell each other exactly what you want—or to be told. It's often really useful to talk about all this afterward.
- **Take sex off the table:** Paradoxically, one of the best things you can do for your sex life is to make it clear when sex is not an option. (This works especially well when you have that shared understanding we talked about in the previous section as to how often you'll actually make love.) That way, you don't have to wonder what that hand on your hip means, maybe starting a downward slide of resisting his affection and slipping into a quarrel. You can enjoy the caress for what it is without fearing what it might become. Couples learn to send these signals gracefully, through hints, subtle shifts in the body, little jokes,

or even straightforward statements like, *How about some hugs before we go to sleep?*

- **Put parts of your body off-limits:** Similarly, you need to be able to declare certain parts of your body off-limits at certain times. For example, some couples have nights when the erotic zones are not to be touched; besides giving each person—well, usually the mother—the sense that her boundaries are respected, it can build an erotic charge for the occasions when the red light turns to green. This ban may become semipermanent for many months, such as in the case of a nursing mother who really does not want her breasts touched by anyone besides her baby.
- **Touch more in bed:** You spend about a third of your lives under the covers with each other, and that's a great opportunity for affectionate touching. Now that you've got some clear boundaries, try to get rid of any pillows between you in bed—and maybe the pajamas as well. If you're using bedclothes as a kind of barrier, or a way to discourage sexual interest, your words alone should be sufficient. If they're not, that's the real problem, which should be addressed through methods more direct than a nightshirt (see the two previous chapters). Lying skin to skin under the covers can feel really safe and nice.

Romance. Remember the little romantic things you used to do for each other? All those gestures were a way to say, *I cherish you apart from all the jobs you do for our family.* As a relationship continues, it is normal for romance to decline, becoming a more everyday love. But when romance disappears entirely, it can start to feel like the principal basis for your relationship is that you are both yoked to the same plow.

Since caring for young children can get pretty unromantic—such as wiping tops or bottoms—try to talk with your partner about what feels romantic to do or to receive. This applies to small gestures such as a love note, roses, and dressing up and to big events such as a special date. Both of you could describe a romantic experience you'd like—and one that is realistic these days—and then make sure you actually do each of them. If you're like most couples after children, there's currently so little romance that a tiny effort will lead to a giant increase.

Erotic affection. The territory between a quick kiss and sexual intercourse often shrinks to nothing after children, with parents acting like asexual, functional partners except when they make an appointment to be lovers. But lacking those little moments of juicy contact sprinkled into your day is a loss in its own right, plus sex without that foundation can feel scheduled and dutiful at best. Further, when there has been a certain juiciness in the air, the partner who's more eager for lovemaking often becomes less insistent about it since some of his or her needs are being satisfied in the ordinary course of your life together.

The key is to have an understanding about erotic touching—about when, where, and how—that works for both of you. You just have to talk about it, respect the sexual natures you each have, and find a middle path. Each of you can stretch a bit. Maybe you'd like a passionate kiss every day that doesn't implicate you in going any further. Maybe he'd like a little fondling in bed at night and be delighted and grateful to receive this pleasure and then drift off to sleep.

Going all the way. Here are some suggestions for the practical problems parents often need to get out of the way before they can go all the way.

- **The child's in the bedroom:** This is one of the prime physical obstacles to intimacy, especially when your children are babies. One mother described her solution for this problem to Ricki: *It's the last thing you think would happen, but our kid has improved our sex life. She's made us be more creative. We* *put her down in the family bed, and then make love in the living room, her bedroom, even the bathroom—places we never would have thought of before.* Other parents find ways to make love discreetly with a sleeping baby in their room.

- **You might be interrupted:** Some disturbances can't be helped: If a sleeping baby wakes and starts crying, you just have to smile at each other in resignation and then tend to your child. But you can prevent other interruptions through a bit of planning, like letting a child stay up a little later to be sure he'll sleep soundly. Or get the kids out of the house altogether by arranging for a friend to watch them or hiring a babysitter to take them to the park (maybe "while we work on our taxes").
- **There's never any time:** There's always *some* time. For example, when the baby goes down, run into the bedroom.* Don't turn to housework or returning calls. Help each other get into it, and soon you'll be glad you did.
- **Your vagina seems "stretched out" after childbirth:** Usually, after a few months, the vaginal walls return to near their original shape and elasticity. If not, Kegel exercises often help, and if they don't, consult your gynecologist.
- **Intercourse is painful for you:** Painful intercourse is normal for up to a year after childbirth, and the lowered estrogen that comes with breastfeeding can leave vaginal walls dry and easily irritated. But it could also be due to a yeast infection or other physical causes, so be sure to mention this problem to your gynecologist. On your own, try longer foreplay, using a lubricant, and slower and gentler movements with your partner. If these methods don't seem to be enough, talk with your gynecologist since there are many good options for treatment.

---

* Just kidding about running. When our kids were little, it was more like staggering.

Addressing deeper issues. Other issues are a matter of the mind rather than a practical problem. If, deep down, there's little natural inclination toward sex, look at the previous section on developing more desire. Otherwise, here are some suggestions:

- **Fertility procedures have complicated sex:** The medical interventions and sex-on-the-clock aspects of fertility procedures can rock a couple's sex life for many years. Check with your doctor and perhaps do some testing to make sure there aren't any lasting effects of hormone therapy on estrogen, testosterone, or other hormones that regulate sexuality. With your partner, you could deliberately retrace the early steps of your romantic relationship, re-creating the freshness and passion that are the best antidotes to any mechanical quality that has crept into your sex life.
- **You're mad at each other:** If it's a spat that day, try to talk it out before lovemaking. But if there continues to be an open sore in your marriage, you can use the methods we've described to deal with it inside yourself or between you. In particular, try to speak about any hurts in your sexual relationship, such as thoughtless comments about changes in your body or disdain about one partner's (high or low) interest in sex. If you can't resolve these issues on your own, we recommend you consult with a therapist.
- **Something traumatic happened during pregnancy or childbirth:** Invasive procedures or insensitive professionals can leave scars on the mind that linger. The passage of time and just talking about it with your partner or a friend can really help. If that's not enough, contact a therapist since there are effective methods for dealing with psychological trauma.

- **Issues unrelated to being a mother are complicating your sex life:** For example, abuse during childhood, rape, or sexual humiliation can lead to intrusive images, feelings of panic or shame, intense dislike of one's body, an abhorrence of sex, or other complications of sexual relations. If any of these might apply to you, it's really worth seeing a therapist.
- **You feel embarrassed about how you look:** If you feel your body is too heavy, or not shaped the right way anymore, try to remember that if he wants to make love with you, it's because you are sexually attractive. Even more to the point, he's probably more excited about making love with *you*, the person inside, than he is about having sex with your body; the most thrilling moments for most men are when their partners are passionate. When that happens for you, he is really not going to care about those stretch marks, or any other detail about your body. If you share your concerns with him, there's a very good chance that his response will be reassuring.
- **It's been a while since you had sex:** You may feel nervous about making love again if it's been a while; sometimes a year or more can pass since the last time a couple with children had intercourse, especially if the woman was pregnant during that period. But you were able to have sex before, and you will surely succeed at it now. Take your time when you make love for the first time again, and tell each other what you need to feel comfortable.
- **Motherhood and sex don't seem to mix:** Our culture tends to draw a double yellow line between maternity and sexuality. When you look inside, can you find any beliefs like that? If you do, you can talk back to them inside your own mind (using the methods outlined in chapters 2 and 3), or examine and challenge them with a friend. Try to let yourself feel how your

physical and emotional fertility as a mother are integrated with your sexuality in one beautiful tapestry.

- **It's hard to shift gears:** Even with a moderate sex drive, most women have to make a conscious transition from mom mode to lover mode. If you think lovemaking might be on the agenda, maybe he could get the kids to bed while you take a warm bath. Perhaps changing into something other than an old flannel nightgown helps put you into a certain frame of mind when you're headed for bed. Or take a shower together or give each other a brief massage.

  When you're tired or afraid the kids will wake up any minute, it's natural to skip the hors d'oeuvres and jump to the main course. Sometimes it's the entrée or nothing, but try to linger with foreplay whenever you can, an important way to warm up and shift into being lovers. You could also spread foreplay throughout the day, building a pleasant buzz between you.

- **It's no longer spontaneous:** Well, so what? Many pleasures, from dinner with a friend later tonight to a pleasant walk next Saturday, are increased through anticipation. Rather than resisting the way that sex necessarily becomes more scheduled after children, see if you can use that to make it even more exciting. If you're planning to make love Tuesday night, you could build up to it with sexy hints, teasing and pulling away *(Wait 'til Tuesday!)*, writing little notes that suggest what you'd like to do, or simply playing with mental fantasies. Aiming for a certain time for sex can help motivate you to be nice to each other and stay out of wrangles. And if you can, try to be open to spontaneous sex at least occasionally, even if it's not really the perfect moment.

- **Sex is boring:** On top of the general issues that can make sex more prosaic as the years go by, becoming parents adds new ones, including diminished libido, less opportunity for anything creative, and a weariness that leads to plain vanilla sex. To rekindle some zest, you could start by thinking about or writing down a list of things you would like to try or change in your sex life, and be as specific as possible. Next, make a second list of the reasons it's hard to suggest these to your partner; when you can look at them down on paper, you'll probably see that most or all of the reasons don't hold water: They're nothing more than the familiar collection of general inhibitions on asking for what you want, or embarrassment or shame about sex. Understandable and normal as these thoughts are, you can let go of them like any other beliefs that dampen your well-being and the quality of your marriage.

  Then, unless you truly believe it would be risky in your relationship, try being very candid about what you like. Just talking about it can be a turn-on. Over time, if you can give each other at least some of what's being asked for, that could make lovemaking very satisfying again. You could also do a variation of the giver-receiver exercise described under "Experiment with affection" back a few pages, this time focused on pleasuring each other sexually. If you like, you could try this two ways (on different occasions), one in which you take each other to climax, and the other in which you get as close as possible and stay there without going over the edge.

  Perhaps read some books, alone or together, about sex in a long-term relationship. Sex is many things, but one of them is that it's a skill that anyone can get better at—like any other skill—through a little study, attempting new things, and practice: a skill that involves the mind even more than the body.

The most profound way to revitalize a sexual relationship is both the simplest and the scariest: It is to open up more, *emotionally*, while engaging erotically with each other, from lingering looks to all-out lovemaking. Sex is so revealing that it is natural to get into a kind of role or script about it as a way to keep feeling safe: As the clothes come off, a subtle mask often comes on. But to be really open while all the intensities of sex tremble inside, exposed to the eyes and touch of your lover, is incredibly exciting. It makes sex fresh again, every time.

Because love is the most tender of the intensities of sex, it is both the most thrilling and the most tempting to hide. For many of us, it is easy to be sexual, easy to be loving—but hard to be both at the same time. Nonetheless, in daily life, the seeming domain of love alone, can we sometimes open the gates of sexuality inside, letting the tingle of eros be present between us as we make a meal together, hand off a child, or say goodbye on our way to work? Or, when being sexual, can we open wide the gates of love? Then we touch with a cherishing in lips and fingertips, the giving of our bodies opening our hearts. Now raising children together adds to our love life instead of subtracting from it: We feel warmed by appreciation for each other, our sexuality an inherent part of the circle of love that is our family.

PART FIVE

Managing the Marathon of Motherhood

Motherhood is a long journey, a marathon, not a sprint. It begins before your first child is born: that incredible moment when you know you've conceived a new being, the long pregnancy, fixing up the baby's room, finally the birth itself, and then the little breathing bundle, the life delivered into your arms. The details differ a bit if you've adopted a child, but the essentials are the same: anticipation, nervousness, and an extraordinary love.

Some parts are a blur, and others a long, slow grind. Feedings, diapers, long nights with the baby, the first steps, the first words, the first everything. Tantrums, story time, bouncing a ball, wiping a chin, high chairs, tiny chairs, wiping crayons off chairs. Day care, preschool, the first day of first grade, watching that sturdy back trudge down the hall to class. Summer camp, Cub Scouts, Girl Scouts, bullies, buddies, soccer games, Little League, balls caught, dropped, kicked, and lost. Chores, bedtimes, discipline, loud voices, angry voices, soft words, loud silences. The grades tick by, good teachers and bad, science fairs and spelling lists, too much homework or not enough, that great moment when your child knows the answer to a question . . . and you don't. Somewhere in there your youngest turns eight or ten and you think, it's half over, where has the time gone? Middle school, high school, pimples and makeup and dating and fingernails chewed after midnight until you hear a step at the door. Strange music and stranger frien[illegible]oltish and gawky, solemn and wise. All the while, the birthdays have ticked by, some with numbers that echo: 1, 2, 6, 10, 13, 16. Then the 18th: What now?

The marathon doesn't end there, though it becomes more meandering and less consuming. Loans that are really gifts, advice that is rejected loudly and followed quietly, graduations, postcards from Mexico or Maui, a down payment with your name on it, walking down a wedding aisle with a grown-up child on your arm and coming back alone. If your children have children, your journey takes on a second sort of mothering. You age and your children don't seem to. There comes that time when the trajectory of your life is clearly falling back to earth as your children's ascends. You drift into old age, and there is a subtle shift of care and power. And then the final moments come, your veined and aged hands in the strong ones of your children, squeezing, a kiss, a final blessing, a farewell, an ending to the path you walked as a mother, and the beginning of a mysterious new one.

It's a long, long road. That's why it's so important to have a few good tools for the practical problems that make your journey harder than it really needs to be. We've seen one bunch of problems, in particular, wear on women year after year: those involved with juggling home and work. In the next chapter, we'll look at how you can solve them.

CHAPTER NINE

Juggling Motherhood and Work

Many women need to balance motherhood and work. Obviously, mothers "work" at home as well as "work" for pay in their occupation, but for simplicity, we'll use the word *work* in this section to refer collectively to one's job, career, or business. Many of the points made would also apply to an avocation that has a central place in a mother's life, such as art or a spiritual practice.

Whether you were only able to take the short leave your company offered and are now back at work full time, have gone to a part-time schedule (perhaps switching careers to do so), or work at home, the juggle is never easy. If you don't currently work for pay, the decision not to may have been a complicated one—as could be any return to work down the road. Consider these mothers we've known.

Donna had two daughters, seven and four, and a full-time job as a checker in a supermarket; she and her husband had separated a year after their second child was born. She came to see Jan about a cold that wouldn't seem to go away. Jan asked what her days were like, and Donna replied matter-of-factly: *They're overwhelming. There's no other word for it. Mario has the girls a couple days a week, but one's on the weekend, so your basic day has me up early to get things ready, drop them off at two different day cares, and get to work I hope on time. They're cranky because I have to hustle them along just to make the schedules work. And God help us if one is sick: Is she well enough for day care? Am I a bad person for infecting the other kids? Can I afford to stay home again this month? What if they call me and I have to leave work? There's no one else; I've got no family here. We get home and we're all fried. I can't be the kind of mom I want to be since I'm so tired. I put them to bed and half the time fall asleep with them and wake up groggy halfway through the night with my neck scrunched into a corner of the bed. The whole thing's like a Swiss watch: If every little part works perfectly with every other part, then the day's OK. But how often does that happen?*

Astrid, a lawyer, had planned to return to work a few months after her first child, Sean, was born. But as she put it to Rick when Sean was about six months old: *I just can't. I'm totally surprised I feel this way, but he's so little and I love him so much that I don't want to be away from him. I thought I'd nurse him for a month or so and then wean, but we're still going and it's so important I don't want to stop that either. But all this is creating a problem in my marriage. My husband wants me to go back to work because it's beyond tight without my income. But every day, Sean does something different and amazing, and I don't want to miss that, or have some nanny be the one who gets to see it all.*

Cora was staying home with her two-year-old daughter, Tatiana, but, as she said at a talk Rick gave to a mothers' club: *It's getting old, and I'm starting to feel very restless at home. Put clothes on, take them off. Make a meal, clean up, make it again. We go out for a walk, but no one's around, just us and the birds. I want to go back to work as a dental hygienist, but my husband thinks Tatiana is too young and his family agrees.*

Mandy had received an unexpected surprise at age forty-two: She was pregnant. Now, several years later, she was the full-time mom of a bouncy four-year-old boy, Isaac, having left her career as an art director for an ad agency. She said to Rick: *I feel guilty about it—because being a mom is supposed to be wonderful and all, but I really miss my old job, the bustle of the office, the travel, the intensity, even the deadlines. It was like the world of an exciting color, you know, red. I totally love my son and I'm happy I'm here with him, but I get pretty bored being home all day, like my world has become beige. And me, as well: For example, my husband and I recently had dinner with people from his office. We introduced ourselves, everybody had interesting jobs, and then it got to me. I said I was a full-time mom. They said, "Oh, how nice," and the conversation moved on. During dinner, people asked each other about their work, but no one asked me about raising Isaac. I felt dismissed and like I had nothing to offer. It made me mad.*

Claire worked at home as a freelance writer while raising Tim, just turned six, and Tammy, "age three, going on thirteen." Claire told Ricki: *People say I've got the best of both worlds, but it's more like the worst of both. I get calls at all hours, but especially in the morning since many of my clients are on the East Coast, and everybody needs last-minute changes, so I have to take the calls. I heard Tammy once tell a little boy, "My mom's job is she's on the phone." Tim's in first grade, so that's finally working, but childcare for Tammy is one problem after another. She's in a great preschool, but the day care is expensive (and I miss her, I admit it). So I get her early, but then it's hard to do more than bits and pieces of work, and definitely no calls: Try talking to an editor while your child keeps calling "Mommy"!*

Problems like these are so commonplace that it's natural to take them as a given. But until the last hundred years or so, motherhood and work were usually woven together with most women working with their young children nearby. While we couldn't say more strongly that mothers have the right to work for pay—or emphasize the fact that fathers could just as readily stay home with children—it remains that the modern division between motherhood and work is completely unnatural.

Yes, the industrialization that's driven these changes has brought many benefits—such as safer childbirth or phone calls to kids who've gone off to college—but one of its costs has been an unprecedented tension in the lives of many women between two callings. If she works for pay, she could miss her children. Yet if she doesn't, she could miss the income, camaraderie, and fulfillment of work.

So if you're feeling pulled in two directions, the first step is to let go of any guilt or self-blame: The tug-of-war between family and work is a modern invention, and none of it is your fault. Nor should it be all on your shoulders to fix or solve or bear—as it's construed so often, both in the media and across the dinner table—since it's a father's job just as much as it is a mother's to balance the need to have bread on that table with the needs of vulnerable young children to receive the attentive, ongoing, and loving care of someone who adores them.

> *The work world has evolved as if employees had no families.*
>
> Marcia Killien, RN, PhD

In the swirl and press of raising a family, in the middle of a society that is breaking new ground each day, you can feel pressured to make quick decisions, go along with the views of a persuasive person or group, or simplify complicated matters by fastening upon one compelling "reason" for one choice or another. But that usually leads to a shaky foundation. Plus often there is no choice at all: You just *have* to do one thing or another.

If there is at least a little flexibility in your options, in the next few pages we'll analyze their major pluses and minuses and see how they fit with your deepest purposes in life and the needs of your family. Then, no matter your situation—related to a job, schedule, or childcare—in the next sections we'll explore ways you can make it work for you.

PLUSES AND MINUSES

Much research has been done on these topics, but even with all the knowledge in the world, you still have to thread your way through a messy bunch of trade-offs.

For instance, studies have found that mothers who work are healthier than mothers who do not.* Sounds simple, right? But behind that headline, there's a messier truth. Research findings are always about the *averages* of groups.† Yet you are a person, not an average! If you read a statement like "Mothers who work are healthier than those who do not," you might conclude, reasonably enough, that you will be healthier if you return to work. But the statement really means only that "The average mother who works is healthier than the average mother who does not." In fact, many mothers who do not work are healthier than many mothers who do. The crux is always individual: What's right for *you*, and *your family*, in *your particular situation*? Let's look at the details that have to be considered to come up with the answer.

Benefits of Working

The many rewards of working start with the enjoyment and fulfillment you experience from the work itself. There could be the feeling that you are using an important capacity within yourself, like a technical or managerial talent. Working offers the satisfaction of accomplishing a specific ambition (e.g., to be a teacher), and some lines of work give you

* However, this apparent benefit is inflated by other factors: For example, women who work are likely to be better educated—which is associated with better health practices and less illness. They also tend to be more healthy in the first place, since people whose health is precarious are less likely to seek work.

† We're using the word *average* as a shorthand term for the various statistical measures of the central tendencies of groups.

the sense that you are making a contribution to society beyond your family. Certain jobs or careers also have prestige or social status. Last and usually not least, there's the additional money a job brings. Bringing home a paycheck can help you feel that you are on an equal footing with your partner and give you more say in how money is spent and the family is run; of course, in principle a relationship could still operate that way when the mother doesn't work.

There are also pluses for the children of a working mother. Some of the physical or psychological health benefits she enjoys from working will spill over onto them—like her feeling more fulfilled, or less likely to have her patience worn understandably thinner from being home with a young child all day. A second paycheck means more money to buy them things, like better food and health care, enriching experiences, and vacations. Then there are future benefits to a child if his mom works when he's little: By not stepping off the career track—especially the fastest ones—she will probably have a larger salary when he's older.

Costs of Working

Now comes the other side of the balance sheet: The benefits of working need to be netted against its costs. Physically demanding work—involving heavy lifting or exertion, or standing on your feet all day—has been associated with poorer health in mothers, especially during the first year after giving birth. Jobs that offer the employee little say in when and how specific tasks are done, especially low-level clerical positions, are a risk factor for cardiovascular problems in mothers. Moving from physical to mental health, you could feel uneasy, worried, or even upset at being separated from your child. Or guilty, perhaps, at not being the sort of mother you want to be.

If nothing else, working means getting to spend less time with your child, and sometimes missing special moments or milestones like the first steps. To have as much time as possible with her children, an employed mother typically sleeps 5 or 6 hours a week less than a stay-at-home mom. Working also means spending more time in traffic (unless you work from home), with the aggravations and expenses of commuting.

Meanwhile, the hassles of investigating, managing, or changing childcare usually land on the mother, and as the difficulty of arranging for childcare rises, a mother's health tends to decline. Once everything is set up and work looks like clear sailing, your job still gets disrupted when a child is sick or needs to be taken to a doctor, and your partner can't or won't handle it. And if you are already heavily burdened—such as by a colicky baby who keeps you up at night or by personal health problems—a job could be the proverbial straw that breaks your back. Adding it all up, it's not surprising that full-time employed mothers of infants report greater stress than do full-time homemakers with infants, and they often neglect their own health to cope with their total workload.

Of course, mothers differ, and a benefit to one could be a cost to another. For instance, some women have the temperament for zooming between a demanding job and a couple of young kids—and in fact, they may prefer to be highly active: Stress for them could be a weeklong vacation with nothing to do. But for others, that sort of life would be highly stressful and depleting, with both short- and long-term impacts on their health and well-being.

In terms of effects on your family, going to work usually means needing to find places and occasions to pump breast milk if you have continued nursing. This is a major reason why returning to work (especially full-time) usually leads a mother to wean earlier than she otherwise would, which means losing the benefits of breastfeeding. Nursing is (most of the time) sweet and satisfying for both mother and child. Besides the intangible benefits for you, continuing to breastfeed seems to help shield you from the effects of stress. And the benefits for your children include a boost in IQ and fewer illnesses—some of the reasons why the American Academy of Pediatrics and the World Health Organization recommends exclusive breastfeeding for the first six months and continued nursing for two years or longer if desired by both parent and child.

For the family as a whole, mornings and evenings get especially frenzied when both parents work. At the beginning of the day, everybody zooms around, getting dressed, packing lunches, and schlepping kids to childcare. At the other end of the day, you've got to shove *so* much into a small sliver of time: hugs and kisses for children, questions like *How did it go at preschool? Was Camila nice to you today?*, and housework tasks that get pushed into the evening or weekend. When—finally—you get the kids to bed, and the last dishes done or the laundry folded, it's hard to have much energy left for yourself or your relationship.

Adding to your stress, kids are often cranky from long hours in childcare and more frequently ill from exposure to other children who are sick—and this brings us to the complex, sometimes touchy subject of the impact of childcare on kids. Some research has found that *moderate, high-quality* childcare, especially past the first birthday, has—on average—some benefits for language development without disrupting the attachment relationship between a typical parent and child, though it does seem to make many kids somewhat more aggressive. But the actual childcare the majority of kids in America experience is completely different: It lasts for many hours each day, sometimes 7 a.m. to 7 p.m.; it is performed—often by one adult for four to six children—by well-intended but usually poorly trained, poorly educated, and poorly paid staff with high rates of turnover; and it starts when children are just a few months old. Plus, the research instruments used to assess potential psychological injury to children cannot fully measure many subtle issues, such as a person's lifelong capacity for a deep, trusting intimacy. Then, even if one assumes there is no injury to a child and no lasting impact, there is still the matter of suffering: Most young children do not like being separated from both their parents. Finally, research on childcare may not apply to your own child, who may be more sensitive or vulnerable than some other kids.

Our point here is not to make anyone feel guilty about using childcare. The options are very limited for most parents, and if you need childcare, you pick the best setting possible and try to compensate for less-than-perfect childcare in other ways. It's simply that childcare needs to be used with a sensitivity to the possible impacts on your own, unique child, for her sake as well as yours.

Summing Up the Benefits and Costs

If you do have some choices, the sensible way to think about work and motherhood is to consider different options—Work or not? Full- or part-time? This job or that one?—in terms of *this* mom with *this* child and *this* partner in *this* family with *this* childcare possibility at *this* time. Let's suppose a mother, Jane, is debating whether to return to work or to continue staying home with her toddler, Sebastian, and big sister Gianna. If Jane is bored out of her skull staying home *and* Sebastian is easygoing and would adapt quickly to childcare *and* her husband is up for doing more housework *and* Gianna is doing fine in preschool *and* there's a good home day care site just down the street *and* Jane already weaned Sebastian months ago, *then* returning to work could make more sense than staying home. But what if the opposite were true? If Jane feels deeply satisfied with being a full-time mom *and* Sebastian is anxious and clingy *and* her husband works very long hours *and* Gianna is jealous of her brother and wants a lot of time with Mommy *and* Sebastian is still nursing, *then* staying home could make more sense.

To be sure, in real life the case for one option or another is usually a closer call: Suppose Jane is climbing the walls at home and her husband is fine with doing more housework, but Sebastian is anxious about separation and the childcare options don't look very good. The needs of children must be balanced against the needs of their parents, who have rights, feelings, and wants that count, too. Even when you consider only the child, there are still trade-offs: Sometimes a "cost" to a child (such as adequate but less than optimal childcare) in one area will be balanced by an even greater gain to the child in another area (such as a mother's greater patience because she is less stressed). Complicating things, there are the trade-offs between present costs and benefits and future ones: Perhaps Sebastian will be quite stressed by Jane working at this time, but he'll benefit in a few years from the additional income and seniority she'll have from continuing to work.

Overall, these are often tough decisions, and whichever way Jane goes there will be problems. But the right decision for any mother, whatever it is, will be the one that considers all aspects of her situation—and then evaluates them in light of her *purposes* and *priorities* in life.

Using Purposes and Priorities to Inform Your Choices

Clarity about your purposes and priorities makes it much easier to make fundamental decisions about working or not, and to inform daily choices. Say your boss offers you a plum assignment, but it entails a week or so of business travel each month. If you know that your priority right now is maxing time with your family, and you're deliberately treading water in your career, then you'll feel more peace of mind about turning down the opportunity. On the other hand, if you've decided to put more energy into your career, you'll feel easier inside about telling a child that Mommy has to go on a business trip for a few days, but she'll be back really, really soon. When you have a clear direction in life, you don't have to continually reevaluate your choices, or agonize over the ones you've made. It helps you deal with people who are questioning, sniping at, or resisting the choices you've made; you know what you feel in your heart, and you're more able to explain your actions (if you need to). Looking deep inside to name what you truly care about centers you, and it enables you to make wiser choices with less stress.

Even if you can't fulfill an important purpose right now, or be entirely true to your priorities, clarity about what's awry helps you let go of self-blame, feel entitled to mourn what's missing, and be motivated to work on creating a life structure that's a better fit with your values.

So how do you come up with your essential purposes and priorities? Just like one sort of job might suit you but not another person, some ways of establishing your purposes will speak to you while others will not. Therefore, here's a sampler of different methods:

- Imagine that you're nearing the end of your life. What do you want to make sure that you are glad about, in terms of the choices you have made? What do you want to make sure you don't regret?
- Consider what you love doing: *What are my passions? What situations or activities make me very happy?*
- Reflect on your moral commitments: *What do I care about deeply? What larger cause do I want to serve? How do I want to make a difference?*
- Consider how improving your condition or capacities in some regard—such as remedying physical depletion, or cultivating psychological growth and wisdom—could be the catalyst or foundation for many positive things. Perhaps that form of personal healing or development should be a priority for the next few years.
- Think about the people you admire, your role models, and your heroes and heroines. What are their characteristics or

actions that inspire you? What might you like to emulate, in your own way, about one or more of these people?

- If this is meaningful to you, you could ask God or whatever is spiritual for you for guidance as to what you're meant to do with your life in general, or with regard to work at this time.
- Make a collage from pictures and words cut or torn from magazines. You can do this on poster board or on individual sheets of paper in a notebook. The theme could be very broad, such as your purpose in life, or quite specific, such as how you want to transition back to working half-time.
- Ask your partner what he thinks your priorities should be at this time. He may have a fresh angle, but don't be overly swayed; the heart of the matter of purpose is what's in *your* heart.
- In one sentence (present tense), try to state your overall purpose in life. It's not set in stone, and you can have a different purpose later on. Some examples: *My family is healthy and happy, and so am I. I live a life of health, happiness, and contribution. My life is an expression of Radiant Being. I am love, communication, and aliveness. I leave the world a better place. I live with integrity, humor, love, and grace.* Also, try to state your purpose as a *mother*.
- Consider how the priorities of family and career may not be in conflict, but could serve each other. For example, being successful at your job could be an important model for your children. Similarly, creating a solid, loving foundation at home could help you feel secure in venturing forward in your career.

Once you've clarified your purposes, take a little time to acknowledge the trade-offs that are inherent in any choices you've made or will make. You can't have more of one thing without less of another, and we've never known a perfect arrangement of home and work for any mother.

Next, we suggest you step back and take a long, honest look at your life. Start by asking yourself where you are living true to your purposes. Let yourself feel really good about that. Then, big breath, ask yourself where you are not. When you reflect on any gaps between ideals and actions, consider first whether it is possible, in fact, to close them. Maybe it's just not possible right now: Perhaps your family simply can't manage without your paycheck, or no matter how much you want to get back to your career, a chronically ill child needs you at home. If you can't pursue some important purpose at this time, the best you can do is to be compassionate with yourself about this, reach out for support, and keep trying to figure out how to fulfill your dreams.

On the other hand, maybe you *could* actually accomplish your purposes to a greater degree. Then it's really important for your well-being to try. If the problem is external, like no transportation to get to work, you could look into ride sharing or other jobs that are closer to bus lines. If it's internal, like feeling too shy to contact people you once worked with to ask if they know about any jobs, you could use the techniques in chapters 2 and 3 to work on that. Usually there's some action, internal or external, that will give you a jump start and get things rolling. For instance, a shy person could invite her former colleagues out for a casual lunch, and then, once the ice is broken, she could steer the conversation to her going back to work and see if they have any ideas.

Above all, seek the balance of family and work that will be truest to your nature, rather than conforming to what other people think. Perhaps you've run into one-size-fits-all thinking in the form of social pressure to work or to stay at home. Advocates for either side can talk as if there's just one natural way to be, and selectively use scientific studies to make their case. But in truth, there is wide variation among women in their natural interest in mothering and working. One of Rick's clients had to muster up her courage to tell him: *I feel really bad about saying it, but a lot of the time, taking care of my daughters is really tiresome and irritating, and I just want to get away. There's no doubt I love them. But when I hear other moms go on about the bliss of motherhood, that's just not me. I have to work, or I'd go crazy—and that wouldn't be good for them, either.*

On the other hand, a different mother (who used to be a stockbroker) was laughing gently at herself one day in Rick's office: *About a month before I was due with my first child, I sent out a letter to my clients saying I'd be back full-time after six weeks, not to worry. But I just fell in love with the little guy, and something completely changed inside me. What had I been thinking?! There was no way I could be away from him all day and leave him with people who could never love him the way I did. Forget it! So we cut back, I stayed home, and I can hardly believe it, but now, several years later, I've become gripped by being a mother and fulfilled in a way I never imagined was possible. I can see a time ahead, maybe when he's in grade school, when I'll want to work again, but that's a ways off, and when it comes, it'll be natural.* The shape of your nature—as individual in its contours as a baby's footprint—may not fit neatly into the hole defined by one cultural model or another, and trying to jam it in or act like there's no friction would just stress you—and, ultimately, your family.

MAKING IT WORK TO STAY HOME

If you've decided to stay home full- or part-time, let's assume that you're using the skills of inner competence discussed in chapters 2 and 3 to manage your stress, stay as relaxed as possible, and take in all the delicious rewards of this time. Your partner needs to appreciate that your role is not a piece of cake and to be helpful in the evening when he gets home. Perhaps most important of all, you need community, especially with mothers. That's what will break up the monotony of your day, give you emotional support and a helping hand, and satisfy the tug in your heart for the company of other moms.

With these as a foundation, let's look at some practical steps:

- **Leave your work mind behind:** Just like a job calls for a whole set of skills and attitudes, so does full-time child-rearing, which has totally different activities and priorities. You just can't care for children and home like a day at work.
- **Use your work skills:** On the other hand, there's no sense in forgetting the work skills you've got that could be useful at home, such as breaking a big task into smaller ones, creating policies, and putting things on a calendar.
- **Take it easy when you can, and let yourself really enjoy this time:** No doubt, there are hard parts of staying home with children. Meanwhile there are all the wonderful moments, too. Some mothers feel guilty about savoring these, as if they ought to be suffering the whole time, like everybody else is (supposedly) at work. But while caring for children, you probably handle situations that are harder than anything most people deal with in a day of work, so when you get a chance to put up your feet and relax, grab it—and linger. You don't have to keep the house spotless or prepare a fabulous meal every night in order to justify your (supposed) "vacation" as a homemaker: It's not a vacation, as anyone well knows who has taken care of children all day. You earned this time with your kids, and it won't last forever. Finally, you *need* to rest and even laze about during the few times each day when you actually get the chance, in order to settle back down the stress chemistry in your body and nurture your health and well-being.
- **Manage the boredom:** For us, the most unpleasant part of taking care of children all day is that it is sometimes really, ah, *boring*. You do the same laundry, work the same puzzle, clean the same counter, read the same book, play the same

game, over and over. That's when the desire to do *anything else* gets especially intense. But what has worked for us and other parents we know is to pay *closer* attention, noticing tiny details you'd normally overlook. This makes the activity suddenly more interesting, and draws you into a more peaceful, contemplative awareness. Similarly, by putting your awareness into your body and releasing any tension or discomfort you find, you'll feel more comfortable and less eager to be somewhere else.

It also helps to look for the nice parts in an activity, or nudge it in a more playful and stimulating direction. For example, you could goof around by putting puzzle pieces in upside down, and see what your toddler does. Or make up a song while she puts them in the right way.

- **Find respites:** Make sure to get some relief from interacting with your child every day. The possibilities include your partner giving him a bath while you read a good book or watch some TV, another mom coming over with a child that will play with your own, or formal childcare. In particular, study the conditions that drag the needle on your internal stress meter into the red zone, like more than a few hours alone in your home with an oppositional three-year-old, and do everything in your power to change them so you never "redline" with stress.
- **Nurture your sense of worth:** To the extent that your job gave you a sense of accomplishment, status, or worth, staying home means finding other sources of self-esteem. The first place to look, of course, is your role as a mother: It's the plain truth that you are making an extraordinary contribution to your children, with results that are visible every time you look at them, and the honor due you for that is magnified by any personal sacrifices you've made to be a mother.

Widening the circle, you could get involved in your children's activities, such as by becoming a room parent in preschool, soccer coach, or teacher in Sunday school. Besides being an excellent way to meet other moms and families, it would add to your sense of making a difference in the world. These benefits apply to other forms of community service as well.

For other suggestions on maintaining your sense of worth, look back at chapter 3.

- **Check in with yourself:** Keep paying attention to how it's really going for you. Are you feeling isolated? Is there a frustrated sense of the world passing you by? If you try some of the previous suggestions and you still feel something important is missing, it could be a sign that you need to shift gears, perhaps by returning to or increasing your work.

MAKING IT WORK TO WORK

The foundation of maintaining some well-being while working is the same as if you were at home full-time: solid stress-relief skills, support from your partner, and community with other mothers and families. On top of that, here are some practical actions you can take to have working work for you:

- **Managing maternity leave:** The Family Medical Leave Act (FMLA) requires businesses with 50 or more employees to give women 12 weeks of unpaid leave, but many companies are not affected by the FMLA, and those that are vary in their individual policies. Make sure you are crystal clear on the details that apply to you, keep a copy of the employee manual or any other applicable records, and take written notes of relevant conversations with a benefits manager or your boss. Once you know what you're dealing with, try to make a plan that's as flexible as possible, because there's a lot of inherent uncertainty about how you will feel and how it will go with your baby, especially if you're a first-time mom. You don't have to give in to pleas or pressure from people at work to return sooner than you'd like: Just keep listening to that wise voice inside you that knows what's best for you and your family.

- **Continuing to breastfeed:** As we've seen, there are many benefits to you and your child of continuing to nurse while going off to a job. In some cases, you could nurse her at your worksite (through on-site childcare or a nanny bringing her to you), zip over to see her if you live (or she's in childcare) nearby, or just go down the hall if you work at home. But more commonly, breastfeeding while working means pumping at work. Unfortunately, most workplaces are at best unhelpful when it comes to pumping, without any place more private than the women's restroom, and some are downright hostile.* Happily, many resources can help you continue with breastfeeding while you work, from trusted online resources to the La Leche League. A lactation consultant (your OB/GYN, midwife, or pediatrician can refer you to one) can advise you about pumping or storing breast milk. Finally, it's important to feel encouraged to continue breastfeeding—by a partner, other mothers, and hopefully coworkers—and if it's appropriate, you could ask for the support you and your baby need.

---

* Besides stressing mothers, this attitude is short-sighted from a strictly business perspective. For example, one study found that working mothers who pumped breast milk had lower absentee rates than other working mothers who weaned their babies (due to fewer colds and other illnesses in their children that required them to come home).

- **Standing up for your rights:** If you feel that you are being discriminated against at work due to being a mother—such as unreasonable exclusion from certain meetings, career opportunities denied, or outright demotion or firing—you can contact the National Partnership for Women and Families for guidance on understanding your rights.
- **Stopping work from spilling over onto home:** The occasional text or call from the office is one thing, but it's another to have already limited time with your children and partner interrupted and consumed by work. You may need to create a polite but firm boundary. Even without the phone ringing, if you're preoccupied by a problem at work, it could help to talk about it briefly with your partner, perhaps blowing off some steam, so you can set it aside for the next day.
- **Working at home:** But what do you do if you work *at* home?! Millions of employees now work remotely at least part-time—many of them mothers—and many other moms run home-based businesses. To stay both relaxed and productive, make it clear to your children, friends, and partner that when you're home, you're still in worker mode and need to have your time and focus of attention respected. But don't let work fill your home like a bad case of Bermuda grass: Schedule specific times to be on the job, and keep work materials in specific places, like inside a home office or on a particular desk.
- **Stopping home from spilling over onto work:** If there's something you really need to pay attention to during the day, like the status of a child who may be too sick to stay in childcare, then so be it: Make discreet phone calls or give your manager a heads-up that you might have to take a long lunch or go home early.

  But if it's one of those common but more diffuse problems—like wondering why your four-year-old still has a case of the terrible twos—you could make a mental appointment with yourself to think/worry/plan about it at a specific time that day, like during lunch, or at your desk for 15 minutes (no one has to know what you're pondering). And do what you can to have your partner handle a big piece of the problem himself: Maybe it makes more sense for him to set up an appointment with a doctor, or make a few calls to start the ball rolling on getting a different babysitter.

Some worksites are friendly places where people feel quite open about their personal situations, whether it's grousing about the commute or comparing notes to see whose child is the pickiest eater. But some aren't so chatty, and it's prudent to err on the side of caution because—unfair as it is—it's not hard to stir up doubts about a woman's capacity to focus on her job if there are any issues with her children. You can always choose to explain something in the future, but once you've spilled your guts about a problem at home, it's all out on the table and there's no way to unsay it. Besides, it's your private life. If you've got to leave to handle something, you can give a brief explanation and then catch up as best you can later. That's all anyone can do.

- **Shifting gears from work to home:** When you get home or to the childcare center, perhaps wait a few minutes to clear your mind, go for a short walk, or just relax. Walking up to your front door, imagine that you are placing any job worries into a basket outside your home, where you can retrieve them on your way to work in the morning—if you really want to. When you first see your children, whether at day care or in your living room, try to let them have your full attention for at least 15 minutes; once they've had that recharge of mommy-juice, it's usually easier to slip away for a bit to change clothes, flip through the mail, or make a quick call.

- **Getting help from your partner:** When you're going off to work, you *really* need a partner who does his share at home. While fathers whose wives work tend to do more than fathers whose wives are full-time moms, working mothers still typically do more total household and child-rearing work than their husbands. If you feel your partner should pitch in more, try the techniques in chapters 6 and 7. You could also tell him that researchers have found that dads who help more with caring for children have greater well-being than dads who do not.
- **Helping kids feel connected to you at work:** If you are taking a baby or toddler to childcare, you could tell him how much he's in your thoughts and your heart while you're at work, and how he can feel your love inside him all day long; in a mysterious way, he may get the gist of what you are saying, and he will certainly sense your care and love.

  With a preschooler, you could make sure he has a photo of you at school (maybe of you working). You could also tuck a picture or note into his lunch box each day, and perhaps call to check in, as long as that doesn't make him upset. You might arrange for him to visit your workplace, maybe on a day when things are least hectic. Look for chances to explain what you do, tell stories about coworkers, or describe the physical setting of your job. You could take pictures of your workplace and perhaps some of your coworkers to show him. At night, you could have your child imagine a glowing, golden rope connecting him to you throughout the day; in the morning, remind him that whenever he wants, he can feel that golden cord joining you together.

- **Picking up signals:** Keep your radar out for signs that two parents working is taking a toll at home, like a toddler who's getting increasingly clingy, or a five-year-old becoming quiet and withdrawn. For the sake of your children, some changes may be necessary if they're doable, such as your partner coming home earlier or you starting work later. Both of you might have to give the kids more one-on-one attention every day, no matter how tired you are. For a reality check, estimate how much time daily *each* kid receives from *each* parent that's *child-centered* (following the child's interests, and not task-focused, correcting, or scolding). If you know in your heart that it's not enough time, you and your partner should make some adjustments if it's at all humanly possible: Besides being good for your child, it will prevent problems that will take even more of your time in the future.
- **Learning from others:** Over the years, many women have blazed trails for working mothers. At your job, there may be other mothers who can mentor you about the ins and outs of juggling home and work at your company.
- **Saying goodbye to "Supermom":** It's hard for a working mother to avoid the traps of feeling that she has to go overboard at home to make up for having a job, or to be a superstar at work to make up for having a family. Sure, it's important to do what you can to stay on top of the details at work or home. But it's almost impossible to avoid some stuff slipping through the cracks. Most of us need to accept the fact that we cannot be outstanding in each of two separate areas, in both our career and our parenthood. Still, a person can be outstanding at the package of the two: *outstanding at being a parent who works.* When you redefine your overall job description that way, it's

a challenge you can actually succeed at. Sometimes an excellent performance in the *total* job requires doing less at work or at home. Or saying no, even if that means disappointing a coworker, spouse, or child. Or making a special effort to nurture yourself in one setting—such as by connecting with others, slowing down, taking breaks, or focusing on activities you enjoy—so that you can excel in the other, year after year, throughout the marathon of motherhood.

AFTERWORD

The most immediately effective ways to take care of yourself are personal, such as eating nutritious foods, and that's why we've focused on them in this book. But no one raises her children in a vacuum, and we need to acknowledge the impersonal forces that stress and deplete mothers.

For example, poverty, injustice, and war strain and frighten families worldwide. The persistent devaluing of women and their work, notably raising children, burdens mothers emotionally and financially. Sweeping changes in the social environment in which humans evolved to raise families have eroded the community support that once lightened the load and lifted the spirits of a mother.

Therefore, the proper care of our precious children is, fundamentally, a *societal* issue. A nation that truly protected and supported its mothers, its families, and its marriages would value child-rearing in its deeds, not just its words. It would have policies like those found in many countries, such as paid family leave, subsidized childcare, and community property laws in the case of divorce. It would strongly encourage fathers to have a major role in the care of young children and to pull their weight at home. In the broadest sense, it would protect the world its children will inherit through preserving peace, justice, and the environment.

This vision of a nation that nurtures its mothers is not idealistic, but hardheaded pragmatism. Yes, the work of mothers is moral: tending to vulnerable children whose beings are entrusted to our care. But it is also highly practical: raising young people to be productive members of society, creating the "human capital" that is the basis of progress and prosperity. A country fulfills its ethical obligations to its children, as well as makes a shrewd investment in its future, when it spends the time, the money, and the caring to nurture its mothers.

Whenever we nurture ourselves, are kind to another person, support organizations that help families, or otherwise contribute to a safe and peaceful world, we take a stand for such a society, and ripples spread out from our actions. If enough of us take those stands, our country and this earth will become a better place to raise children, and to be a mother.

APPENDIXES

APPENDIX A

Defining Depleted Mother Syndrome

When a mother's depletion is long-standing, severe, and harmful to her health, we propose that she has depleted mother syndrome (DMS).

WHAT IS A SYNDROME?

A syndrome is a group of signs and symptoms that occur together and can help predict a person's prognosis and guide her treatment. Examples of syndromes include premenstrual syndrome (PMS) and acquired immune deficiency syndrome (AIDS).

A syndrome is typically not as well defined as a "disease" or a "disorder." It can be caused by more than one thing, present a variety of symptoms, take a varying course, and respond to more than one treatment. And it can incorporate several individual disorders within its overarching umbrella. For example, a person with chronic fatigue syndrome may have arthritic conditions and insomnia, as well as fatigue itself. Similarly, a woman with DMS may have nutritional deficiencies, sleep disturbance, infection in her digestive tract, and depression—each of which is a health problem in its own right. The various elements of a syndrome appear together because they have underlying causes in common, or they lead to each other.

In sum, we suggest that maternal depletion and its correlates form a coherent whole, organized in self-perpetuating ways, that is a diagnostically distinct and meaningful condition.

Diagnosis of Depleted Mother Syndrome

DMS is defined as *a biopsychosocial condition in which the combination of a mother's outpouring, stresses, vulnerabilities, and (low) resources drain and dysregulate her body.* Specifically, we propose the following criteria for a diagnosis of DMS:

1. *History of outpouring, stress, vulnerabilities, or low resources related to raising children.* Indicated by the combination of:
   - **Outpouring:** Such as two or more pregnancies, or extended nursing
   - **Stress:** Such as raising young children, caring for a child with a challenging temperament or a health problem, or serious conflicts with her partner
   - **Vulnerabilities:** Such as history of trauma, preexisting physical or mental health problems, or a reactive or sensitive temperament
   - **Low resources:** Such as poor nutrition, little chance for rest, minimal help from her partner, little care of children by others, or lack of community
2. *Drained nutrients.* Indicated by laboratory findings of low levels of important nutrients, such as vitamins, minerals, amino acids, or essential fatty acids.

3. *Dysregulated systems.* Indicated by signs and symptoms that one or more of the following systems are significantly dysregulated: gastrointestinal, endocrine, nervous, or immune.
4. *Rule out other medical conditions.* The drained nutrients or dysregulated systems are not caused by another medical condition (although other medical conditions may coexist with DMS).

Individual Variations

DMS can vary from woman to woman in terms of its severity, duration, and course.

Differential Diagnosis

Postpartum depression. The standard definition of postpartum depression (PPD) is that it is a major depressive episode that begins within 4 weeks of delivery and is resolved within 6 to 12 months after delivery. DMS differs from PPD in several ways:

- DMS is based on physical depletion (which is not part of the definition of PPD).
- The symptoms of DMS do not necessarily include depression.
- DMS often appears a year or more after the baby has been born, because of the gradual accumulation of depletion.
- DMS can linger long after the first year postpartum.

The "maternal depletion syndrome." Several years after Rick coined the term *depleted mother syndrome*, we found references to a "maternal depletion syndrome" suffered by malnourished women in lower income countries who frequently bear and breastfeed multiple children with short birth intervals. DMS differs from maternal depletion syndrome (MDS) in two regards. First, we use the term *depletion* to refer to specific, moderate to severe nutritional deficiencies in an otherwise reasonably well-fed person, while in the context of MDS, depletion generally refers to an overall condition of (sometimes extreme) malnutrition. Second, our definition of depletion includes disturbed bodily systems; MDS focuses on nutritional shortages. In essence, DMS is a broader and milder condition than MDS, and it is rooted in the social context of higher income nations. Clearly, we were not the first people, by any means, to be concerned about the depletion of mothers. Whether the construct of DMS can be applied in Third World settings far removed from our professional experience remains to be seen, and we offer it respectfully for consideration by scholars and professionals working in that area.

APPENDIX B

A Safe Room in Your Mind

This exercise should take 10 to 30 minutes, depending on how deeply you get into it, so try to do it when you won't be interrupted. You can use it for expressing your feelings, thoughts, and desires. If you are getting more upset, not less, please immediately stop the exercise and shift to doing something calming and soothing for yourself.

THE EXERCISE

Find a comfortable place to sit or lie down. Close your eyes and take a minute or more to relax your body.

Visualize a completely safe room, either one that is familiar or one from your imagination. Make it as real as possible by visualizing the details, such as thick walls, a strong door, or a force field around the entire room. Keep deepening your sense of the utter safety of this room. You are completely in charge of it. Only you can decide what can come in. You have total control over what happens in the room, and you can decide at any time to send something back out.

Experiment with bringing a completely safe, supportive person into the room, perhaps someone you know or even an imagined being such as an angel of light. See if that helps you feel even safer and stronger. But do not yet bring in anyone who is challenging for you.

When you are ready, let yourself experience some of the feelings you want to release. Keep remembering that you are utterly safe and secure, that you have complete control over everything that happens in your safe room, and that you can increase or lower the intensity of the feelings as you choose.

Then express your feelings in whatever way works for you. You could imagine saying them softly, firmly, or loudly—or in a hurt, anxious, sad, or angry tone. You can scream your head off if you like within the safe room in your mind. You can also imagine yourself expressing emotion symbolically through pounding on the floor, tearing things apart, breathing fire, and so on.

Perhaps that alone will feel complete. If not, you could bring the person(s) that your feelings may be related to into your safe room. Remind yourself that you have complete control within this space, and then imagine the person in the room with you. Make him or her as real in your mind as you are comfortable with. Knowing that you have complete control over what happens in your safe room, you could ask the person to be willing to hear your feelings; inside this room in which you have complete control, imagine that they tell you they are willing and notice how that feels. Alternately, you could skip this step if you like and just start communicating.

Being aware of what would be helpful for you, you might imagine that the other person is immobilized and must listen to you as long as you want to talk. You might imagine them as being very small compared to you, perhaps on the floor while you stand above them. You could imagine them staying quiet or perhaps speaking, even in a loving way. You can express yourself any ways that are helpful for you, softly or loudly, with hurt or love or anger, and perhaps physical contact from hugging to hitting and everything in between.

You can ask the person questions, and listen to what he or she says. Or you can have the person say things that you need to hear.

Throughout, stay focused on what will be most valuable for you. For example, communicating in order to experience letting go is probably better for you than communicating in order to reinforce and intensify your sense of upset. See if there is anything more to express, especially deeper, more vulnerable feelings or wants. When you feel a sense of completion or that you simply need to move on, finish up your communications to the person for now. You could imagine that the other person has really heard, really received what you had to say. If you like, acknowledge the person for being with you. Then send him or her out of your safe room.

You can repeat this process with other people, or communicate with several people at once. You can vary the format and bring individuals into your safe room without first venting by yourself. And you can have the supportive beings in your room say things to you or to the other person. See if you can find an intuitive wisdom inside that knows what will be most valuable for you to do, and also what your limits are.

You can completely let yourself go in your safe room. But there is a fine line between releasing an emotion and intensifying it. If you find that your feelings are getting stronger rather than dissipating, shift to a different mode within the exercise. Try expressing them more softly, sincerely, vulnerably. Or reach for the softer feelings under the harsher ones. Be gentle with yourself, especially if you have had any seriously distressing or traumatizing experiences. You can do this exercise again and again, if necessary, emptying the bucket of painful feelings one spoonful at a time.

Complete the exercise by seeing if there is anything else you would like to communicate, either into your safe room or to any supportive beings that are with you. Thank the supportive beings for their presence, and see if there is anything they have to say to you. Acknowledge yourself for making an effort and being brave. Notice how you feel. Relax even more deeply and let any uncomfortable feelings drain out of you. Focus on positive feelings and let them grow and fill you. End the exercise by saying a kind thought for yourself or brief prayer. Then recall the actual room you are in, rub your hands on your thighs and your feet on the floor, and open your eyes.

AFTER THE EXERCISE

Take a few minutes to let the experience settle before getting up and going about your day; you might like to do something relaxing at first, such as taking a shower.

APPENDIX C

A Mother's Suggested Daily Values

Nutrient	Standard DV	Pregnant DV	Lactating DV	MSDV	Intensive Daily Dose (IDD)	Comments
Vitamin A	2,300 IU	2,500 IU	4,290 IU	5,000 IU		Do not exceed 5,000 IU of vitamin A if you are nursing or pregnant, or for several months before pregnancy.
Vitamin B1	1.1 mg	1.4 mg	1.4 mg	30–50 mg	50–500 mg	
Vitamin B2	1.1 mg	1.4 mg	1.6 mg	30–50 mg	50–500 mg	
Vitamin B3	14 mg	18 mg	17 mg	30 mg		At higher dosages, use niacinamide to avoid flushing.
Vitamin B5 (Pantothenic acid)	5 mg	6 mg	7 mg	50–100 mg	500–1,000 mg	
Vitamin B6	1.3 mg	1.9 mg	2.0 mg	50 mg	50 mg pyridoxine or 50 mg of P-5-P	P-5-P = pyridoxal-5-phosphate
Vitamin B12	2.4 mcg	2.6 mcg	2.8 mcg	200 mcg	2,000 mcg sublingually, 1–3x a day	

Nutrient	Standard DV	Pregnant DV	Lactating DV	MSDV	Intensive Daily Dose (IDD)	Comments
Folic Acid	400 mcg	600 mcg	500 mcg	800 mcg; 1,200 mcg if pregnant	800 mcg; use a methylated folic acid	
Vitamin C	75 mg	85 mg	120 mg	1,000–3,000 mg	2 g up to bowel tolerance	Divide into 2–3 doses taken over the course of the day.
Vitamin D	600 IU	600 IU	600 IU	400–2,000 IU	5,000 IU until a vitamin D test is fully normal	
Vitamin E	22 IU	22 IU	28 IU	200–400 IU	800 IU	Try to get a supplement that has a variety of tocopherols (including gamma) and tocotrienols.
Vitamin K1	1 mg	1 mg	1 mg	1 mg		
Vitamin K2 as MK7	90 mcg	90 mcg	90 mcg	90 mcg		
Vitamin K2 as MK4	5 mg	5 mg	5 mg	5 mg		
PABA				50 mcg		
Biotin	30 mcg	30 mcg	35 mcg	500 mcg		
Choline	425 mg	450 mg	550 mg	500 mg		
Inositol				500 mg; 250 mg if pregnant or lactating		
Beta-carotene				20,000 IU	100,000 IU	Consume as mixed carotenes in your foods, or as high-quality supplements.
Bioflavonoids				500 mg		
Coenzyme Q				60–100 mg		
Calcium	1,000 mg	1,000 mg	1,000 mg	1,000 mg		Try to get calcium citrate, malate, or hydroxyapatite.

Nutrient	Standard DV	Pregnant DV	Lactating DV	MSDV	Intensive Daily Dose (IDD)	Comments
Chromium	25 mcg	30 mcg	45 mcg	400 mcg		Try to get chromium picolinate.
Copper	0.9 mg	1.0 mg	1.3 mg	2–3 mg	1 mg per 15 mg of zinc	
Iodine	150 mcg	220 mcg	290 mcg	300–400 mcg		
Iron	18 mg	27 mg	9 mg	18–30 mg; 60 mg if pregnant or lactating	Up to 60 mg if iron deficient on lab test; 30 mg taken twice daily	Best from organic liver; or take supplements of ferrous glycerinate, succinate, or fumigate.
Manganese	1.8 mg	2 mg	2.6 mg	10 mg		
Magnesium	320 mg	360 mg	320 mg	500 mg; decrease if diarrhea occurs	400–800 mg; decrease if diarrhea occurs	Try to get magnesium citrate, malate, or glycerinate; magnesium glycerinate helps avoid diarrhea.
Molybdenum	45 mcg	50 mcg	50 mcg	500 mcg		
Potassium				2–5 grams from food		This amount from supplements would be dangerous.
Selenium	55 mcg	60 mcg	70 mcg	200 mcg	400 mcg	
Zinc	8 mg	11 mg	12 mg	30 mg		
Omega 3 Oil as fish oil containing approximately equal amounts of DHA and EPA	1,000 mg	1,000 mg	1,000 mg	1,000 mg	2,000-4,000 mg	
Omega 3 Oil as flax oil				1 tablespoon	2 tablespoons	

APPENDIX D

The Insider's Guide: Finding the Right Practitioners and Procedures for Your Unique Health Care Needs

The prospect of going out and finding good care for your health problems can seem pretty overwhelming, especially if you are in the throes of DMS. It can be so tempting to listen to one person who gives you hope, close your eyes, and jump. But the days of the all-knowing doctor who had the time to get to know you thoroughly, while staying current in the latest research on every single modality within the spectrum of care, are long gone—if they ever existed at all. Your health will probably do best over the long run if you work with several good professionals, check out different approaches and weigh their evidence carefully, try cautious experiments, and set your course based on your own experience.

So, where to start? How might you go about choosing practitioners and approaches that are best for you? Let's begin with four key guidelines.

FOUR GUIDELINES FOR NAVIGATING WITHIN THE SPECTRUM OF CARE

1. **Do no harm:** The more sensitive your body has become, the more it makes sense to start treatments at low levels, intensify them slowly, and consider modalities that have the least likelihood of side effects (such as Energetic or Dietary). On the other hand, we need to avoid the harm of using a weak or worthless intervention; this is the principal risk of alternative approaches, and one of the reasons why a physician should always be a member of your health care team. For example, Jan has seen several mothers attempt to treat their low thyroid problem with nutritional supplements alone when, in retrospect, they should have consulted with a physician about a prescription. We think you should routinely get good assessments within the framework of Western medicine both to help with maternal depletion and to identify any other health condition you may have.

   It's also important to avoid the harm of treating symptoms while overlooking root causes. For example, many women have recurrent vaginal yeast infections that they treat topically—time after time—without ever addressing the underlying conditions that predispose them to these infections, such as a weakness in their immune system. The root causes of an illness commonly include stress and lifestyle factors (such as not exercising, or abusing alcohol), and you can improve these with the methods discussed in parts 2 and 3 of this book. A general imbalance or weakness in one or more systems of the body is frequently another fundamental source of illness—especially subclinical, chronic conditions—and these are often helped by alternative approaches.

2. **Use methods with good evidence:** You'll often hear about some new treatment that's being trumpeted loudly—or seemingly debunked. It might benefit you (or not, if it's been dunked in debunking), but how do you know what's really true? With the internet, you can look up research on health topics by going to PubMed (PubMed.ncbi.nlm.nih.gov). Judicious use of AI tools can also be helpful—including using a second tool to check the work of the first one.

   The chance that something will work for you increases as the evidence for it comes from sources higher up on this list:

   - Careful meta-analyses of dozens or hundreds of studies
   - Multiple, high-quality studies that converge in their findings
   - One double-blind, randomized study with a control group
   - One so-so study
   - A professional's clinical experience with many patients
   - Preliminary indications that an intervention might help based on an understanding of the workings of the body
   - Anecdotes about one person's response to an intervention

   Nonetheless, much medical information today—particularly about innovative or alternative interventions—comes from sources below the top two above.* For example, many of the practices used day to day in Western medicine have not yet been evaluated in multiple, high-quality studies. And alternative treatments have generally received even less research (though European studies are often quite sophisticated), since most of them cannot be patented and thus pay

* Unless otherwise stated (e.g., "We've seen . . ."), the interventions we suggest are usually based on at least one study.

back the costs of careful studies. This means that their potential benefits are more *uncertain*, but it does not mean there is certainly no benefit: As the saying goes, absence of evidence is not evidence of absence.

Sometimes the evidence for or against some intervention will be very solid. But often it will be more uncertain, especially when you consider more innovative or less-studied methods. For example, a methodological problem often occurs in those studies on nutrients that do not find a significant benefit, because many of these do not screen their subjects to see if there is a nutritional deficiency in the first place. If numerous participants already have high levels of the nutrient, they will usually get little benefit from supplementing it—thus reducing the *average* benefit and perhaps making it appear that the nutrient has little to offer, when in fact it may have considerably helped those subjects who began the study with low levels. It would be like doing a study on Prozac in which a substantial fraction of the participants already were receiving moderate doses: The average impact of the drug would appear reduced.

There's really no way around it: We all have to make decisions about our health care in which we weigh the odds of the potential benefits and costs. If the risks of an intervention are low—such as with most of the alternative modalities in the spectrum of care—then it may well be worth trying even when the evidence for its benefit is mixed, but if the risks are relatively high, then you should have stronger indications that it's likely to help.

3. **Work with the right people:** It's important to look for people who stay within their own area of knowledge while respecting

the work of other professionals within the spectrum of care.* For example, few holistic practitioners have a deep understanding of the pharmacology of Western medicine, yet some might tell you not to take a prescription drug. Similarly, few physicians are trained in nutritional work, yet some might tell you to throw away your supplements. Whether it's an alternative practitioner or an MD, watch out for arrogance, close-mindedness, dismissiveness, dogmatism, or zealotry. A warning sign is when someone tries to talk you out of doing a certain test; it's one thing to recommend against an *intervention*, but we see little sense in recommending against *gathering information* that may make your health care more focused and effective.

You usually have some options in your health care providers, and if you do not get the support and rational open-mindedness you need, look for other professionals. Many people, including us, use several practitioners for different things: perhaps an HMO doctor handles your annual physical exam or any urgent care, while other licensed individuals have primary responsibility for helping you with chronic, subclinical conditions such as DMS.

So who can help you replenish your body and balance its systems? Many professionals trained in Western medicine can,

---

* Unfortunately, many people have little choice about their health care professionals, usually for financial reasons. On the other hand, some managed care organizations are starting to include alternative methods, and many alternative care providers are relatively inexpensive. You can also educate yourself free of charge on the internet about new options in health care.

including physicians (MDs), osteopaths (DOs),* nurse practitioners (NPs), and physician's assistants (PAs) (the last two work under a doctor's supervision). But ask about their experience with nutritional or functional medicine since these subjects were probably not studied in depth in their formal training.

More often than not, though, you'll have to look to other licensed professionals for many of the methods you can use to reverse depletion. Doctors of Oriental Medicine (DOMs) and acupuncturists (LAcs) are sometimes knowledgeable about biochemistry and nutrition from the perspective of Western science, in addition to their expertise in a very different model. Many chiropractors (DCs) have a strong background in nutrition. Finally, many states have a license for naturopathic doctors (NDs), who receive training in both Western medicine (including pharmacology) and alternative methods (especially nutrition and herbs); if your state has such a license, an ND may be most able to offer the integrated approach we generally suggest.

If you are looking for a practitioner, you could start with asking your friends for referrals; the key words that flag licensed professionals who use an integrated approach include complementary, nutritional, functional, or holistic medicine. Your doctor or your child's pediatrician may be able to give you a referral even if he or she doesn't practice that sort of medicine. You could contact the national or county association of the profession you'd like to work with. Or search more widely online.

---

* These are doctors who have completed medical school as well as received specialized training in the musculoskeletal system.

4. **Revise the approach based on your own results:** A method with good research support could be useless for you or have overwhelming side effects; alternatively, studies might be unable to find a statistically significant benefit for some intervention, but it works wonders for *you*. Methods that were once helpful may stop working, and others that used to do nothing for you could suddenly start making a real difference. Or you may get no benefit at first from a supplement or herb (which often take up to 8 weeks to reveal their full effects)—which over time becomes clearly helpful. In all these cases, your personal experience should be your ultimate guide as you tailor your care to your own, individual needs.

GETTING A GOOD ASSESSMENT

The foundation of effective health care is good assessment. There are many tests available that can help your health care provider target specific imbalances in your body. It's like casting a net into the sea; if the mesh is too coarse or dropped in just one place, you may not catch the important fish you are looking for. Similarly, you need an assessment that is both *fine-grained* and *comprehensive.*

> *If you drag a net with a 2-inch mesh through the sea, you will conclude there is no such thing as a fish that is shorter than 2 inches.*
>
> Arthur Eddington, PhD

Who Does the Assessment

An assessment is only as good as the professionals who do it. There is something about being a mother that inclines some practitioners to offer reassurances instead of information, and then send you on your way. In addition to this "motherism," we know many women who have encountered a health professional who:

- Did not want to order tests that took time to interpret or cost money
- Held the patronizing belief that "all that information will just confuse you" or "it will just send you down rabbit holes of further testing"
- Dismissed findings that did not fit his or her assumptions
- Did not try to figure out complex results
- Thought that very low or very high results were just fine as long as they were within the extremely broad "normal range"
- Refused to look at any lab reports that used colors to highlight key results (!)

It's best to work with people who respect your intelligence, consider health in a comprehensive and holistic framework, actually try to figure out puzzling results, and explain their thinking. Persist in getting your questions answered and the help you need, or find another professional. Standing up to the health care system can feel daunting even on a good day. It may help to have your partner or a friend come along for support.

Several health care providers might manage different aspects of your assessment. If several people are involved, one person, often a physician, should integrate the findings into a coherent picture. A family doctor or gynecologist may be the right person to do this, or a specialist in women's health, but we generally suggest that you try to work with someone who is knowledgeable about good nutrition and optimizing gastrointestinal function—which are key to reversing depletion.

Making Sense of the Findings

Avoiding mistakes. An assessment can miss the boat in two ways. A *false-positive* error occurs when it looks like there's a problem but there actually is not, which can lead to unnecessary treatments with potentially harmful side effects. A *false-negative* error happens when no problem is found but there actually is one, so undiagnosed conditions then go untreated. Depending on the test or medical laboratory, these errors can be surprisingly common. It is wise to ask practitioners about their estimates of the false-positive and false-negative rates in the tests they use. If they resent your question, do not understand it, or do not know how to get some kind of answer, that is a yellow flag about their support for you or their expertise.

Keeping tests in perspective. Laboratory tests are only part of a total assessment. You have a right to speak up if a professional dismisses your concerns and palpable symptoms because of test results that do not definitively indicate a problem. You also have a right to probe the thinking of your practitioner—who, frankly, has probably not had much time to analyze your testing, given the time pressures in health care systems these days—or ask questions about what the findings mean, such as:

- What do these low numbers mean? How about these high numbers?
- Why should I worry about how much A or B I have?
- What could be the relationship between X and Y (e.g., low tryptophan and depressed mood, low thyroid and achy joints)?
- Why are A or B so low if I've been taking supplements?

Link current tests to your health history. Health professionals today usually have little time to put current findings in context. Keep a copy of your previous lab reports and bring them to your appointments—especially if the tests were ordered by a different practitioner. Then you can compare current test results to past ones and ask the professional to explain what is getting better—or worse—and *why*.

Compared to what? Many test results are interpreted in terms of where you stand within the *range* of a comparison group. For example, a 5-year-old who can read 500 words would be high within the range of other children her age, but a 16-year-old who can read only 500 words would have a low score among others her age. The group your results are compared to is crucial to a correct understanding of your health status. If the range is skewed incorrectly in one direction or another, then a truly problematic test result may be erroneously considered "normal," which would be a false-negative finding. Therefore, try to ask about the sources of the "reference range" your lab uses. If your health professional or lab does not understand your question, dismisses it, or cannot track down an answer, that's a yellow flag.

In particular, we strongly suggest that you scrutinize so-called "low-normal"* results, especially of nutrients. The "normal range" is typically set between the 5th to 95th percentiles—based on the questionable assumption that 90 percent of the population is perfectly healthy. If your test results fall close to the high or low end of the "normal range," they will be ignored more often than not. We think that's misguided for several reasons. First, the population used for the reference range may not be especially healthy in the first place! For example, if your iron levels were at the 20th percentile of women your age, that might seem acceptable until you consider that the majority of women are thought

* Occasionally, high—rather than low—is problematic; for example, high-normal thyroid stimulating hormone (TSH) may indicate that you have low thyroid. The points in this paragraph would still apply, but with the percentiles reversed.

to be at least a little anemic. Second, low-normal conditions matter in their own right. For example, if your child's academic test scores were in the bottom 20 percent of his or her class but above the 5th percentile, how would you feel if a teacher told you everything was fine? Finally, mothers need extra reserves in their bodies to cope with future stresses, so they should aim for the high-normal end of the range.

We hope that these tools will help you get the care that you—that all of us—truly deserve. Because it probably took many months for your body to become depleted, it may also take some time to start feeling the effects of treatment. But with patience and a willingness to change course when something is obviously not working, you *will* most likely feel better. And if you don't, it's time to try a new approach. You deserve to feel good in your body and full of the energy you'll need for this long and lovely journey of parenthood.

ACKNOWLEDGMENTS

Much as it takes a village to raise a child, it takes another sort of village to write a book.

First and foremost, we must express our gratitude to the many mothers who have been our clients or patients over the years, whose insights, stories, and voices echo throughout this book. We've also learned much from the questions and examples offered by the mothers and fathers who have attended our talks. And we very much appreciate the mothers—Jennifer Abbe, Anne Marie Buckland, Lisa Demarias, Deborah Johansen, Carole Kammen, Janet Lipsey, and Pennie Sempell, JD—who participated in the discussions we held on the topic of community.

Numerous people took the time and trouble to read drafts of the manuscript and offer suggestions, including Scott Anderson, MD; Debra Bell, MD; Shoshana Bennett, PhD; Karla Clark, PhD; Caren Cole, DC; Jenifer Cortwright, MFT; Vicki Darrow, MD; Sarah Ferguson, MD; Nancy Frease, MFT; Linda Gaudiani, MD; Elson Haas, MD; Pam Handelman, RN; Ann Hathaway, MD; Kristin Jokel, Evelyn Kade, LAc; Risa Kaparo, PhD; Rick Martinez, MD; Jim McQuade, MD; Jennifer Bean Parks; Cindy Shearer, DA; Cherie Trombly, MS; Bob Truog, MD; and Shellie Wilkinson. In particular, Deb Moskowitz,

ND, of Transitions for Health, painstakingly reviewed the chapters on physical health and made many important suggestions. And Caroline Pincus provided crucial editing and guidance.

An early version of this book was published by Penguin, where Jenifer Ehman and Jane von Mehren were top-notch editors, ably assisted by Jessica Kipp, as well as warm and humane voices on the other end of the phone who clearly felt a personal commitment to the welfare of mothers and families.

Many other colleagues gave encouragement and constructive criticism, notably Adrienne Amundsen, PhD; Chris Berman, MPH; Michelle Borgault, MD; Nancy Boughey, LCSW; Wanda Bronson, PhD; Carolyn Pape Cowan, PhD; Philip Cowan, PhD; Mary Croughan-Minehane, PhD; Charles Dohlbaum, MD, PhD; June Engle, MD; Leah Fisher, LCSW; Tina Gabby, MD; Rachelle Halpern, MD; Leslie Horn, PhD; Ifeoma Ikenze, MD; John Kells, PhD; Eric Kelly, MFT; Phyllis Klaus, MFT; Jonathan Kopp, PhD; Judy Lane, NPrac; Alicia Lieberman, PhD; Judy Loring, CNC; Melody Lowman, PhD; Kerista Luminiere-Rosen, PhD; Dennis Malone, Kristen Skenfield Marchi, MPH; Sally McGuire, PhD; Rick Mendius, MD; Dayton Misfeldt, MD; Jon Pangborn, PhD; Joan Patterson, PhD; Mary Piel, MD; Jane Rowe, MD; Stephen Seligman, DMH; Richard Shames, MD; Mary Jane deWolf Smith, PhD; Lane Tanner, MD; and Barbara Williamson, CNM. Although there are too many to name, we'd also like to thank all of the doctors and staff at California Pacific Medical Center who generously shared their expertise and resources while we were preparing this book.

Of course, our friends and family have been a vital source of practical help and moral support. They include Nan Bakamjian, Melba Beals, Judy Bell, David Boulton, Lynne and Jim Bramlett, Tom Bowlin, Rosalie and Jim Clark, Roberta and Jim Cummesky, Daniel Ellenberg,

Keith Hanson, Raven Jones, Dan and Joy Millman, Leslie Patton, Terry Patton, Michelle Rivers, and Mike and B. J. van Horn.

More broadly, we are indebted to the work of thousands of researchers and clinicians in the fields of clinical and developmental psychology, nutrition, obstetrics and gynecology, Chinese medicine, and alternative and complementary medicine. Further, as parents and as professionals, we have benefited from the feminist scholars and advocates who have greatly improved the health and well-being of women and mothers.

Renee Brna has been an extraordinary researcher, editor, and young mom herself whose craft, diligence, feisty finickiness, and cheerful can-do spirit are woven into every page.

Our agent, Amy Rennert, is the perfect balance of kindness and practical wisdom, and she made many suggestions that dramatically improved the writing in the book. And Stephanie Veillon—our dear friend, the CEO of Being Well, Inc., and mega mama—has been the crucial foundation for doing this book at all.

Last and far from least, BenBella has been truly amazing to work with. What a great combination of professionalism, competence, reasonableness, and sincere passion for the subject of this book! We are very grateful to Sarah Avinger, Kim Broderick, Kellie Doherty, Madeline Grigg, Ariel Jewett, Alicia Kania, Adrienne Lang, Lindsay Marshall, Claire Schulz, Clara Tamez, Susan Welte, Karen Wise, and Glenn Yeffeth.

Thank you, everyone!

INDEX

ABOUT THE AUTHORS

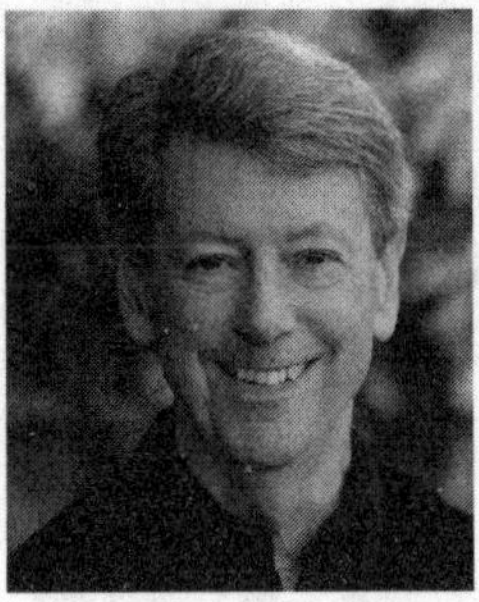

Rick Hanson, PhD, is a psychologist, senior fellow at UC Berkeley's Greater Good Science Center, and *New York Times* bestselling author. Altogether, his seven books have been published in 33 languages and include *Making Great Relationships*, *Neurodharma*, *Resilient*, *Hardwiring Happiness*, *Just One Thing*, *Buddha's Brain*, and *Mother Nurture*, with over a million copies sold in English alone. He's the founder of the Global Compassion Coalition and the Wellspring Institute for Neuroscience and Contemplative Wisdom, as well as the cohost of the *Being Well* podcast, which has been downloaded over 25 million times. He offers free newsletters, and his online programs have scholarships available for those in need. He's lectured at NASA, Google, Oxford, and Harvard. An expert on positive neuroplasticity, his work has been featured on CBS, NPR, the BBC, and other major media. He began meditating in 1974 and has taught in meditation centers worldwide. He and his wife live in northern California and have two adult children. He loves the wilderness and taking a break from emails.

✧ ✧ ✧

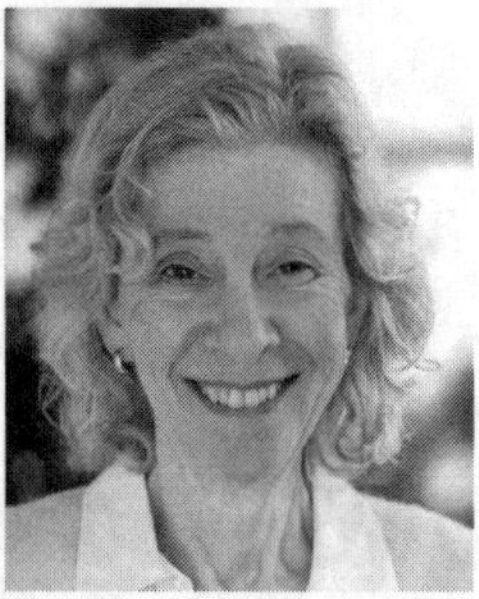

Jan Hanson, MS, LAc, is a licensed acupuncturist and integrative health practitioner with more than four decades of experience in nutritional medicine, functional testing, and holistic approaches to well-being. Building on early training in biochemistry, she is one of the early pioneers in bringing evidence-informed nutritional medicine into mainstream complementary care. Jan has taught widely, offering practical guidance on topics such as digestive health, allergies, and women's wellness.

Known for her clear, compassionate teaching style, she has supported individuals and families in improving their health through accessible, step-by-step methods. She lives in northern California with her husband, psychologist and author Rick Hanson, and enjoys time with their two adult children.

✧ ✧ ✧

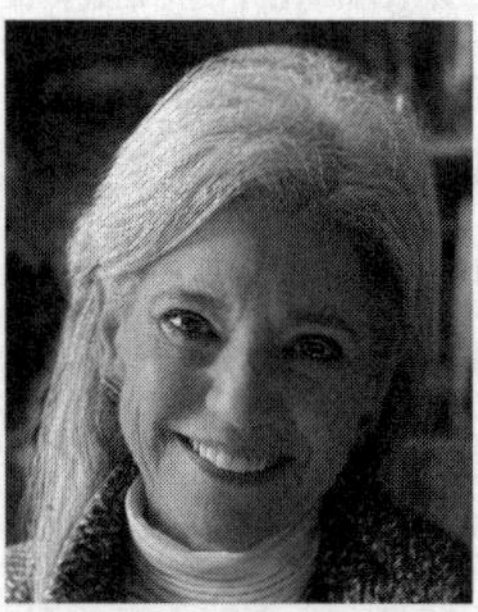

Ricki Pollycove, MD, MS, is a nationally recognized expert in OB-GYN, caring for women through all stages of their lives. She is passionate about helping to optimize health and inspire self-care despite multiple demands in a complex world. She is a mother and grandmother, having delivered babies while also raising her own daughter from age 3 as a single mom.

In active clinical practice for over 40 years, she authored *The Pocket Guide to Bioidentical Hormones* and has appeared on national TV, radio, podcasts, and YouTube videos on fertility, motherhood, nutrition, hormones and mood, breast cancer, perimenopause, and healthy aging. She has authored scientific papers on testosterone, female sexual dysfunction, osteoporosis, and every aspect of menopause. Dr. Pollycove continues to provide medical education to doctors and clinicians worldwide.

✧ ✧ ✧

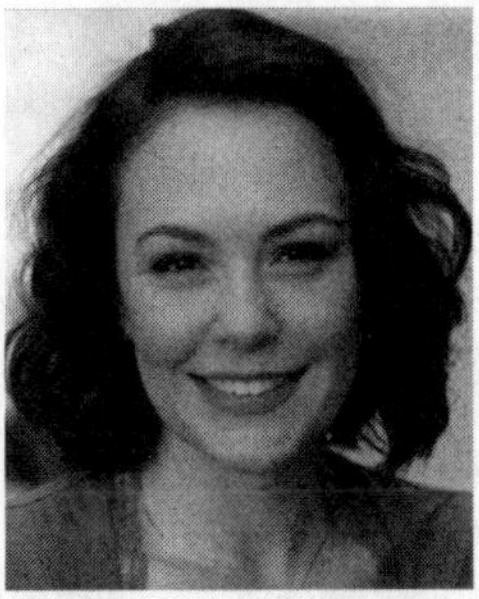

Renee Brna is a clinical therapist-in-training in the marriage and family therapy program at the University of Nevada, Las Vegas. Her work focuses on parental well-being, burnout, and mindfulness-informed approaches to supporting families. She brings experience in crisis counseling, community programming, early childhood education, and psychological research. A mother of two, she first turned to the book *Mother Nurture* by Rick, Jan, and Ricki during her own early parenting years and later contributed new writing and updated research to this book. Before entering clinical training, Renee worked professionally as a Broadway and television performer.